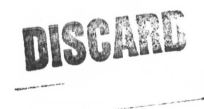

More Than Skin Deep

More Than Skin Deep

Exploring the Real Reasons Why
Women Go Under the Knife

LOREN ESKENAZI, M.D., F.A.C.S.,
and PEG STREEP

*HarperCollins*Publishers

This book is written as a source of information about plastic surgery. It is intended as a reference source only. All readers contemplating plastic surgery should discuss the matter thoroughly with their doctors, and the information contained in this book should by no means be considered a substitute for that advice.

All efforts have been made to ensure the accuracy of the information contained in this book as of the date published. The author and the publisher expressly disclaim responsibility for any adverse effects arising from the use or application of the information contained herein.

The names of certain individuals discussed have been changed to protect their privacy.

Materials in chapters two and four were published in another form in *Consciousness & Healing: Integral Approaches to Mind-Body Medicine,* edited by Marilyn Schlitz and Tina Amorok with Mark S. Micozzi, published by Elsevier Churchill Livingstone in 2005.

FIRST EDITION

Designed by Mary Austin Speaker

Library of Congress Cataloging-in-Publication Data

Eskenazi, Loren.
    More than skin deep: exploring the real reasons why women go under the knife / by Loren Eskenazi, and Peg Streep.
        p. cm.
Includes bibliographical references and index.
ISBN: 978-0-06-057788-9
ISBN-10: 0-06-057788-6
    1. Women–Surgery. 2. Surgery, Plastic. 3. Beauty, Personal. I. Streep, Peg. II. Title.

RD119.E85 2006
617.9'5—dc22

2006045768

07 08 09 10 11 ID/RRD   10 9 8 7 6 5 4 3 2 1

To my dear friend Elizabeth Targ and all the healers who venture into yet-uncharted waters, guided not by clear sight but by intuition, not by definable outcomes but rather by unproven yet nonetheless palpable results. You are bringing the light we so desperately need.

—L.B.E.

CONTENTS

1

Cosmetic Surgery and the Promise of Transformation

Some twenty-five years ago, I went to medical school to become a healer. I chose plastic surgery because the transformation it offered patients was immediate and life-changing. As a young medical student, I witnessed cleft lips made whole, birth defects rectified, and missing body parts re-created, and I fell in love with the extraordinary promise offered by the specialty. I traveled to foreign countries as part of a surgical team that in real and visible ways altered the lives of hundreds of adults and children over the course of a few weeks. I saw that each life and each surgery was unique, and I felt sure and confident that this was medicine at its finest and most personally fulfilling.

Now, having performed roughly ten thousand surgeries and undergone three procedures myself, I spend my days as the founding partner in an all-women's practice in San Francisco, where I devote half my time to breast reconstruction after cancer and half to cosmetic surgery in all its forms. I now see that the healing we offer as surgeons isn't always as clear-cut as it once appeared, and that cosmetic surgery raises questions and concerns I didn't anticipate when I was just beginning.

I've grown troubled as cosmetic surgery increasingly becomes, with each passing year, a commodity in American life, a readily available answer to dissatisfaction with all aspects of the physical self. Where it was once the province of the rich and famous, it's been fully democratized. It no longer needs to be done in Beverly Hills or Manhattan or cost a fortune, and more and more women each year from all over the country are choosing it. Information about procedures as well as local advertising from doctors offering their services are readily available on the Internet, testifying to the ubiquity of this surgery. Type in "cosmetic surgery" on Google and you'll get more than 1.5 million matches.

Each year, more and more American women elect to have cosmetic surgery, and the trend shows no sign of abating. More than 10 million surgical and nonsurgical procedures were performed on women in 2005, and by the time you read this, the number will undoubtedly be higher, as it has been with each passing year—a reflection of cosmetic surgery both as a cultural fact and a phenomenon. It has become a reliable growth business: In a single year—between 2003 and 2004—the number of abdominoplasties increased by 28 percent, the number of breast lifts 19 percent, the number of liposuctions 28 percent. In 2004 the number of breast augmentations went up 9 percent, and the abdominoplasties another 12 percent.[1] This growth shows that cosmetic surgery has become just another product in our consumer society.

These are seismic changes and are having an effect on our culture and how we think about beauty, age, and our bodies. But we don't appear to have developed the philosophical tools we need to understand how these changes can help us live better and more fulfilled lives in the future or how these changes may, in the alternative, make personal happiness more elusive.

I actually had the opportunity to see how quickly attitudes toward cosmetic surgery changed when I participated in teaching a course in biomedical ethics at Stanford University in the early 1990s.

I lectured undergraduates on body modification and plastic surgery for several years, and during that time, I witnessed an extraordinary shift in attitudes. The first year I taught, I asked my students if they would ever consider plastic surgery, and their answer was a resounding "No way!" They were judgmental about people who chose to alter their appearance. The second year, the answer was still a categorical no, but this time, a number of students knew someone who had had surgery and they were mildly curious about the possible benefits plastic surgery could bestow. Astonishingly, by the third year, one-half of the class answered that they would, indeed, opt for surgical improvement, although they remained troubled by how plastic surgery had the potential to install uniform standards of beauty in a culture. By the fourth year, when I asked the question, the class was solidly in favor of cosmetic surgery and said they would absolutely avail themselves of it; their only caveat was cost. In fact, by then, they thought it should be covered by health insurance. For better or worse, young people are more flexible than their elders.

For our children and their children, cosmetic surgery will actively shape how our culture defines feminine beauty, assesses physical "perfection," and responds to the process of aging. In the face of a growing demand for the improvement and refinement of the physical characteristics we're born and age with, my profession will continue to be motivated to seek out new techniques, which will, in turn, bring in more patients. In the future, we'll be seeing the patient pool—now concentrated between the ages of thirty-six and sixty-four, with the majority of women between forty-five and fifty-five—get younger as procedures are performed earlier to stave off the early signs of aging and as "proactive" surgery becomes the norm.

While this should make me feel good about a wise career choice, it gives me pause.

As a woman, a doctor, and a patient, I feel we've reached an important watershed moment. Contradictions abound when it comes to cosmetic surgery. First, for all that Americans seem fascinated by and drawn to the promise of improvement that cosmetic surgery offers, they also believe that those who choose it are weak and insecure. Even as scientific research begins to decipher the complex relationship between the mind and the body, popular culture continues to insist that the mind and the body are separate and that the "mind" is morally superior to the body. What this means in practical terms is that women who choose to have cosmetic surgery for reasons that might be healthy and self-affirming will nonetheless be stereotyped as vain or overly concerned with appearance. As a result, there's no dialogue about how changing the body can and does change the "self" or the mind—even though there is plenty of scientific evidence at hand.

At the same time, there's a dangerous trend in the media to minimize the risks associated with surgery and to de-emphasize the rigors of recovery. In fact, surgery changes us in profound ways that go far beyond the results we see on the surface and should therefore never be trivialized.

So-called "reality" shows such as *The Swan, Extreme Makeover, I Want a Famous Face,* and *Dr. 90210* have contributed to both trends in significant ways. On the one hand, they have brought the promise offered by cosmetic surgery into the American mainstream, but on the other, by presenting it as theater or spectacle with exaggeratedly needy and desperate participants, they have only reinforced the stereotypes of the women who choose it. More dangerously, they suggest that multiple procedures performed weeks apart were actually performed on a single day and carry no extra risk. (Even *People* magazine asked the obvious question in its headline after 10 million people tuned in for the last episode of *The Swan:* "Has TV plastic surgery gone too far? Sixteen women, 151 procedures: Is this a good thing?")[2] Multiple procedures and what I would call "extreme" surgery, which leaves the woman looking nothing like herself, are neither healthy nor desirable, and that is precisely what these shows promote.

The promotion of supposedly "scarless" surgery (which *doesn't* exist) and the "weekend" facelift also contributes to the public's misconceptions, as does the extensive use of "before" and "after" pictures, which suggests both that surgical results are more consistently predictable than they actually are and that recovery is minimal. Research demonstrates that calling elective surgery "cosmetic" has lulled Americans into believing that the surgery being performed is somehow less dangerous, less complicated, and requires less surgical skill than either "plastic" or "reconstructive" surgery.[3] The word *cosmetic* seems to connect surgery with lipstick and hair dye—things you can pick up at a drugstore that are perfectly "safe"—and thus encourages people to think that "cosmetic" surgery entails less pain and a shorter recovery period. Needless to say, "cosmetic," "plastic," and "reconstructive" surgeries are precisely the same in terms of risk and recovery.

I would say instead that elective surgery is an important and potentially life-changing event that should *always* be carefully considered.

Finally, despite America's apparent embrace of cosmetic surgery—the rising number of surgeries, the television programs, the magazine articles, the media attention—our cultural attitudes toward it remain deeply ambivalent. With the sides drawn—those all for it on one side and those against on the other—there doesn't seem to be a forum in the middle for meaningful discussion about what changing yourself through surgery entails.

As I see it, our ambivalence about cosmetic surgery and our reluctance to talk about it openly and directly have three related consequences. First, a percentage of women will continue to have cosmetic surgery for reasons that may be inherently unhealthy but, in a consumer society where cosmetic surgery is just another product, will remain unexamined and unchallenged except for the most obvious of cases. (By obvious, I mean patients with body dysmorphic disorder, who have a history of multiple surgeries and, usually, a history of complaints against their former plastic surgeons—all "red flags" for a doctor. Some of these women will emerge from surgery in worse shape than they were in before.) Second—and this is even more important—the women who actually choose cosmetic surgery for reasons that are self-affirming and positive will be effectively isolated by social criticism and will, in many cases, internalize that ambivalence. This has created a subculture of shame and gossip, which is most evident in the magazine articles and Web sites devoted to analyzing whether celebrities have had "work" done, but affects ordinary women as well. Finally, and most important, as a society we aren't coming to terms with the real ways in which surgery alters more than the surface of the body. Beyond the obvious physical changes it creates, surgery has always been and will continue to be a tool of great power.

What discussions we do have about cosmetic surgery—no matter which side we take—just skim the surface. The opponents of cosmetic surgery dismiss the idea that the transformation it offers could be anything other than superficial; they see women who choose cosmetic surgery as filled with self-loathing, insecurity, and vanity, or the unwitting dupes of a female-bashing and quick-fix culture. In the main, despite the increasing numbers of women choosing to alter themselves surgically, our culture remains distrustful of the impulse for many different reasons. In the end, as research has found, most men and women believe that women who have surgery are "more vain or insecure" than women who don't.[4]

The proponents of cosmetic surgery, on the other hand, downplay the risks and minimize the fact that invasive surgery changes us in ways both predictable and not. They ignore the fact that many of the contemporary images of feminine beauty touted as "desirable" are hardly womanly, healthy, or, in fact, attainable by any means other than surgery, since the number of women born on the planet with oversized breasts and no other body fat can probably be counted with ease. They don't address the cultural double standards applied to aging in women and men. They do not acknowledge that *some* women will seek cosmetic surgery because they are overly focused on their looks, afraid of aging, trapped by unrealistic expectations of what a woman and her body "should" look like, or because of a host of other reasons that are more unhealthy than not. They discount the fact that seeing the body as a "project" that is the "ultimate expression of self"—a pattern discerned by historian Joan Jacobs Brumberg in adolescent girls and young women—isn't good for any woman, young or old.[5]

Discussions about cosmetic surgery, both pro and con, are usually placed in the following contexts: the pressure our contemporary culture puts on women to be young and beautiful; our society's focus on scientific advancement ("If it can be done, do it!"); and our American passion for self-improvement in all its forms. And while these discussions can be interesting and even pertinent, they do little to help women understand the choices open to them or the impulses that drive them to make certain choices.

I've written this book as an "insider"—as a plastic surgeon, a woman, and a patient—to explore in depth what it means to submit to the surgeon's knife and how the outer transformation wrought by the surgeon can be made a part of inner transformation as well.

The Invisible Divide

Both members of my profession and insurance companies have distinguished between "cosmetic" surgery—which is elective and, by current medical standards, not clinically necessary—and "reconstructive" surgery, which is medically indicated. This distinction, present from the very beginnings of plastic surgery, puts reconstructive surgery at one end of the spectrum (considered ennobling, "serious" medicine) and cosmetic surgery, which aims only at improving appearance, at another (considered frivolous, and perhaps not "medicine" at all). There's no question that the distinction is made by ordinary people, too, and supports the underlying cultural suspicion that seeking to change the body by choice reveals an inner weakness or spiritual failings.

Our focus on the "why" of surgery—maintaining the difference between reconstructive and elective surgeries—is an everyday reality in the waiting room of my offices, where it has created an invisible but nonetheless palpable divide.

Furnished in maroons and gold velvets and silks, our waiting room looks more like a living room than anything else, with comfortable and inviting furniture, meant to put my patients at ease. The visual centerpiece of the room is a life-size sculpture of a nude woman, lying on her side. She is curvy and sensuous, and looks comfortable in her own skin.

Sitting on one side of the room are the women who find themselves in my office not by choice but by virtue of their disease. Some of them will be wearing hats, scarves, or wigs, the headgear of life with chemotherapy, and each of them has faced breast cancer as well as a life and a body profoundly altered. Even though our society now understands and validates why these women have sought reconstruction of their bodies as a path to healing their souls, it's worth remembering that as recently as ten years ago, reconstruction after mastectomy wasn't considered "necessary" enough for insurance to cover it. Only the tireless and courageous advocacy of patients and doctors alike changed the cultural vision of what constituted "necessity." For these women, being in my waiting room is a step in the journey toward healing and wholeness.

On the other side of the room are the women who are there by choice and who, most important, do not suffer from an illness. On any given day, these women will represent a cross section of women all over America: women with their small children in tow; women in the prime of life still testing out their life path; women who have raised families and women who have stayed childless; working women and stay-at-home moms. There are thin women and curvy women and blondes, brunettes, and redheads, dressed in everything from jeans and a T-shirt to business attire with pumps. On the surface, what they have in common is that society disapproves of them for seeking something that is deemed unnecessary or frivolous—less cumbersome breasts, a smaller nose, a flatter stomach, a more youthful face, or thinner thighs. Almost all of them have internalized society's judgment, and seeing the women across the room from them doesn't make them feel any better about themselves. When they make their way into my office for their consultation, they will often mention how vain or embarrassed they feel when they see the women who really need my services.

As a woman raised in our culture, I wasn't immune to the forces that created that invisible "do not cross" in the middle of the room. As a patient, I understood it from the inside out and initially chose to tell few people about the procedures I'd undergone for fear I would be perceived as weak, insecure, or vain. As a physician, I acknowledge those patients who, despite technically successful surgery, seemed in the end to be motivated largely by the need to please someone else, whether a lover or a husband or a culture that seems to set the bar higher and higher for a woman to look "good" or young. Finally, I had to ask myself whether I was helping to make the world an easier or harder place for a woman to be self-fulfilled and to love herself. I came to realize that the only way I could answer that question was to listen to my patients with care.

For the last decade, I've started each cosmetic consultation with two key questions: "How long have you considered this procedure?" and "Why have you decided to have it now?" Over time, the answers to my questions revealed a common thread: Almost every patient electing surgery had undergone a major life change within the previous year or was anticipating one in the very near future. The life changes were varied—a birth, a divorce, a death, a marriage, a milestone birthday such as forty, fifty, or sixty, or a significant change in life circumstance—but the decision to have surgery was, I came to see, born out of a need to mark the event or transition physically or to have the outer body reflect an inner change that was already taking place. Although it may seem paradoxical, the majority of my patients use their surgery as an opportunity to heal and grow.

I began to question the divide in my waiting room in other ways. Was it possible that, despite the significantly different impetus for the surgery, the experiences of the surgery itself and its unseen effects were more alike than not? I had been taught to focus on the reason for the surgery as the major differentiation between reconstructive and elective procedures, which permitted me to ignore that the "how" of surgery was a constant for the doctor and patient. As I began to look past that traditional division, I began to see that the essential experience of surgery stayed the same, regardless of whether it was elective or not. I knew that the body and the mind always responded to the invasive nature of surgery, but was it right to assume that the response would be different in kind because the surgery was elective?

As a surgeon, I have seen that healing can, indeed, come out of both kinds of surgery, and while the journey of a woman diagnosed with a life-threatening disease is importantly and radically different from that of a healthy woman, there are also meaningful similarities. This understanding came slowly over a period of years, and required that I cast aside my own long-held ideas as well as the succinct but spiritually empty answers I learned during my years of medical school and training. I began to fathom how the decision to alter one's body was endowed with immense power and agency and how "healing" wasn't a synonym for "cure." My own experiences as a patient and my own concerns about whether I was healing or harming my patients in the cosmetic part of my practice led me to look for answers in more out-of-the-way places than my traditional medical training might have suggested.

If I hadn't been a woman in a largely male profession with largely female patients, if the issues pertaining to women and feelings of self-worth hadn't been important to me, if I hadn't been subject to the same cultural pressures as every other woman, or if I hadn't had a lifelong interest in the connection between mind and body, spirit and flesh, I might never have found the answers I did. Perhaps if my practice had been limited to purely reconstructive surgery, as I naively expected in medical school, there would have been no questions to answer.

Surgery—with its risks, its implicit and explicit surrender of control, its cutting and wounding, its recovery, and the marks and scars it leaves—is central to my understanding, which correlates our contemporary surgical alterations with ancient rites of passage and initiation practiced the world over. Throughout history, humankind has celebrated life stages and passages by marking the flesh, and has understood the alteration of the body as part of a larger spiritual experience that changes the mind or soul. My own realization that all surgery constitutes a rite of passage evolved out of my patients' stories, my own surgeries, and my lifelong interest in symbolism and ritual. And, once I understood this principle, I also saw that the steps of surgery are virtually identical to those of initiation rites.

This book is about the work I do when physically healthy women walk through the door in search of transformation and elect to have surgery. Most of my patients don't choose to have surgery for the superficial reasons that come first to mind but because they are in search of something else more profound. For them, taking on the risk that surgery entails is an essential part of the process of inner transformation, which they have already begun on their own.

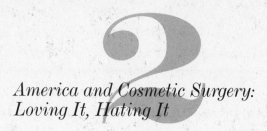

America and Cosmetic Surgery:
Loving It, Hating It

For a country passionately and single-mindedly devoted to self-improvement in myriad forms, the attitude toward cosmetic procedures—whether they are surgical, like a facelift, or nonsurgical, like Botox—is often hostile or, at the very least, ambivalent. It's a river fed by many different cultural streams, some of which date back to the country's European and Puritan roots. Confronting these older ideas is the first necessary step toward understanding why our culture distrusts almost all of the impulses that lead women to choose cosmetic surgery.

Some of the critical responses to the burgeoning interest in these procedures reflect historical and social ideas that have always pertained to cosmetic enhancement—including makeup—and, more specifically, embellishments to female beauty. They form the backdrop to our contemporary discussions about beauty as well as cosmetic surgery, and are so abundant in our culture that they function like the details in rooms we have lived in for a long time, meaning they are so familiar as to go unnoticed. These ideas, not coincidentally, have a long and complicated connection to misogyny in Western thought, since cosmetic enhancement and its supposed corollary, a woman's increased powers of seduction, have been considered suspect since the time of the Greeks. The ninth-century B.C.E. poet Hesiod—who also neatly reworked older myths into the story of Pandora, which made a woman responsible for all the evils and sorrows in the world—warned that the use of cosmetics indicated a duplicitous soul, thereby establishing a point of view with impeccable ancient and classical credentials. Both the Old and the New Testaments paint the corporeal and the spiritual as opposed, and in the Bible's imagery, both personal adornment and female seduction often stand for turning away from God and truth. *Vanity*, after all, means empty and worthless.

In the West, the "fakery" of cosmetic adornment remained a theme with considerable moral and religious ballast up through the beginning of the twentieth century, conflating the image of a woman who used cosmetics with the seductress and the deceiver, the hussy and the vixen. On the other side of the divide was the "good" woman— both natural and moral. As late as 1770, the English Parliament actually enacted a law that dealt with women who had "trapped" their husbands into marriage by other than natural wiles—that is, "by the use of scents, paints, cosmetics, washes, artificial teeth, false hair, Spanish wool, stays, hoops, high-heeled shoes, or bolstered hips." The punishment for those women was nothing less than a witchcraft proceeding and immediate voiding of the marriage. (Spanish wool, by the way, was nothing more than a variety of rouge, though presumably a popular one.)

While the 1920s and 1930s in the United States witnessed the triumph of artifice when hair dye and makeup moved out of the ghetto of prostitutes and "fast" women into the mainstream, the cultural belief in so-called natural beauty held fast, despite the fact that America's women embraced makeup wholeheartedly. It's important to remember that America's fascination with cosmetic surgery started at the same time. Using cosmetics in the 1920s and 1930s became a symbolic act—just as *not* using them in the 1970s would—signifying a new and emboldened view of womanhood. Not surprisingly, many of the arguments against cosmetics were, in fact, arguments about female autonomy and independence in disguise, since the changed status of women was reflected in their use of cosmetics.[1] Arguing about the morality of "putting on a face" was, in fact, shorthand for challenging women's much more public and liberated roles as they stepped out of the home and into jobs and schools of higher learning. In the end, the debate about makeup and cosmetics became the model for our contemporary dialogue about the much more permanent enhancement offered by cosmetic surgery.

Despite the fact that the cosmetics industry in the United States was started by entrepreneurial women for women, the images of beauty presented in the earliest cosmetic ads supported standards of beauty and ideals of femininity that were part and parcel of older stereotypes, as they largely do today. They were visions of the feminine as young and white and, in time, sexual. The promise of transformation was also part and parcel of the marketing of cosmetics in the early years of the industry; in fact, the word *makeover*—now a staple of our culture—was originally coined by *Mademoiselle* magazine in 1936 when its pages featured one of their readers as the "Made Over" girl. "Before" and "after" pictures—now a foundation of our culture of self-improvement, including those used by cosmetic surgeons— were first used as a vehicle for advertising cosmetics, along with the implicit assumption that by changing one's looks, one could change one's life.[2]

But while the female public's wholehearted embrace of the promise of cosmetics (by 1948, 80 to 90 percent of women wore lipstick, two-thirds used rouge, and 25 percent wore eye makeup) would be relatively free of criticism through the 1950s and early 1960s, all of that would change abruptly in the late 1960s, in part because what had begun as businesses run by women for women became, in time, companies run and marketed by men to women.[3]

The influence of the counterculture's emphasis on looking and being natural and the first important feminist criticisms against both the practice of wearing makeup and the male-dominated visions of beauty that promoted it suddenly changed attitudes toward not just makeup but other acts of beautifying the self as well. Beautification, the argument went, was just a manipulation of women's insecurities and their desire to please, and served to keep women under male dominance, both at home and in society at large.

The arguments against makeup would lay the groundwork for the strongest arguments against cosmetic surgery to be leveled some thirty years later. Seen through the prism of feminism, cosmetics—and all other forms of beautification—which incorporated imagery promoted and sold to women by men, were inherently political acts. These arguments, revived with vigor some twenty-five years later in books such as Naomi Wolf's *The Beauty Myth*, would be retooled and refitted as part of the cultural bias against cosmetic surgery, largely practiced by men but largely performed on women.

The history of modern plastic surgery illuminates how this happened.

Out of the Trenches, or Leaving the High Ground

In its modern reincarnation—from the beginning of the twentieth century—reconstructive surgery has always held the high ground, morally and socially. The twentieth century didn't invent plastic surgery—it's been around since ancient times and was part of the field of scientific experiment from before the Renaissance to the nineteenth century—but it didn't come into its own as a possible specialty until World War I, when the doctors and patients were male. Both the numbers of soldiers grievously injured and the type of injuries suffered changed the practice of medicine, and forced rapid innovation and experimentation to deal with the wounded. As historian Elizabeth Haiken notes, both trench warfare and the newly invented airplane left the head and the face of the soldier extremely vulnerable. In addition to other injuries that were the by-product of modern warfare, head and face traumas became the wartime norm, on a scale previously unseen in human history. While modern plastic surgery deals with the whole body, in the beginning, its focus was specific.[4]

Challenged, physicians responded with innovative reconstructive surgical techniques, as well as improvements to anesthesia and antibiotics, that not only healed the individual but made it possible for him to return to society after the war. Then as now, reconstructive surgery had both a physical and social aspect. It reintegrated the body disfigured by birth defect, illness, or accident and, by virtue of correcting those defects, reintegrated the individual into society. In the context of the early history of plastic surgery, "defect" had a relatively tight denotation: outside the norms of health, functioning, and appearance, thus warranting medical intervention. At the beginning—certainly in the first years after World War I—since the specialty was still focused on injury, the definition of "norms" was clear enough. If born out of grim necessity, plastic surgery seemed emblematic of humanity's and medicine's highest and noblest aspirations.

But, in truth, the genie was already out of the bottle. The birth of modern plastic surgery in the first three decades of the century coincided with other major changes in the United States—the ratification of the Nineteenth Amendment, giving women the vote; the invention of the car, the movie, the radio, the telephone; the rise of the modern media; and the birth of psychology and psychiatry, among other developments. These were seismic changes and plastic surgery was part of the rumble. By the time society refocused on the question of what constituted a "normal" and "healthy" appearance, both cosmetic surgery and new connotations for "defects" and "deformities" had already taken center stage, which is where they remain today.

By the 1920s, cosmetic surgery—with both its "life-changing" possibilities and its limitations—was front-page news. In 1923 the beloved Jewish actress and comedienne Fanny Brice had her nose "bobbed." Brice herself offered various explanations for why she'd chosen to alter herself—everything from wanting to look "prettier" to not wanting to be "artistically" limited by her nose (meaning, one guesses, that she didn't want to be a star of just the Jewish theater)—but the more salient part of the story was the public reaction. Her nose job was widely understood in the media and by the populace to be a good and gutsy move; the *New York Times* positively gushed in a 1920s version of today's "You go, girl!" writing, "Hurrah for the intrepid Fannie [sic], whose motto is all for art and a nose well lost." (The witty and acerbic Dorothy Parker, however, dissented from the groundswell of approval, noting that Brice "had cut off her nose to spite her race.") But, in the main, the American audience of the 1920s embraced cosmetic surgery, and the "makeover" gained a foothold in the American imagination.

For those of us who assume that *Extreme Makeover* and the other television shows are a twenty-first-century invention, we may be surprised to learn, as historian Elizabeth Haiken unearthed, that in 1924 a newspaper in New York actually sponsored a contest that promised "the homeliest girl in New York" plastic surgery that would make a beauty of her. The feature ran each day of the month of December—the closest thing to a reality show the times had to offer. Most important, the contest promised the winner total transformation; indeed, as the ad put it, "Here is the chance for New York's homeliest girl. Her misfortune may make a fortune for her."[5]

In many ways, cosmetic surgery was a media phenomenon, and in her book *Venus Envy,* Haiken argues that the linking of two developments of the day—Alfred Adler's theory of the "inferiority complex" and the transformative possibilities of cosmetic surgery—expanded the meanings of "defects" and "deformities" as used by contemporary plastic surgeons and the general public. As she writes, "By the late 1930s, words like 'deformity' had come to connote any and every physical attribute that might spark the feelings of inferiority that would threaten an individual's chances for social and economic security and success."[6] The theme was repeated in magazines and newspapers, as well as in advertising, which embraced many products and services, including soaps, hair products, and makeup. Haiken notes another development important both to the practice of cosmetic surgery and to the public perception of it, as doctors relinquished making "objective determinations about what constituted a deformity" and instead "they listened to their patients' statements about how their faces made them feel."[7]

This was indeed a turning point, and one that continues to affect every contemporary discussion of cosmetic surgery. As the original and tight definition of a deformity that demanded medical attention slipped from view, those physical characteristics that needed "fixing" became a matter of prevailing tastes and subjective points of view—creating a new type of cultural discomfort.

In the first years of the new millennium, America's dual fascination with and aversion to cosmetic surgery reached new heights, even as the number of procedures continued to rise. Writing in December 2002, in a piece with the clever title "The Knife Under the Tree," Maureen Dowd noted that "Santa's sleigh is brimming with gift certificates for the knife, the needle, the laser, and the vacuum pump." The conclusion she drew was caustic and to the point: "It's no longer considered rude to tell someone you love that he or she looks like ten miles of bad road, and suggest major resurfacing. It is no longer important to like people just the way they are; you can like them the way they were and the way they will be."[8] At the same time, the introduction of "reality" shows such as *Extreme Makeover, The Swan,* and *I Want a Famous Face* helped take cosmetic surgery even more mainstream by exposing large numbers of viewers to specific procedures and their possible results on the one hand, and on the other, making even more suspect the motivations of both the patient and the surgeon.

On *The Swan*, a young woman walked down a runway, with a "before" picture projected as a backdrop. There was only a faint resemblance between the slim woman with a mouth full of gleaming, unnaturally even white teeth, wearing a low-cut gown to show off her grapefruit-sized breasts and high heels to accentuate her toned legs, and the image behind her of a frumpy heavy-set woman in baggy clothes, no makeup, and unkempt hair. It's little wonder that the resemblance was so slight since this twenty-seven-year-old had, in addition to a four-month course of extensive physical training and dieting, undergone sixteen separate surgical procedures including a nose job, lip enhancement, a chin implant, a brow lift, a breast lift, liposuction in five different places, and major dental work. Her long hair, too, was a matter of artifice, created by woven hair extensions. Even though Rachel Love-Fraser, a self-proclaimed "ugly duckling" in search of transformation, was declared the winner on the finale of *The Swan* in 2004, she looked amazingly like the other contestants who were all Barbie dolls grown large with exaggeratedly big breasts, nipped waists, big lips, cheek implants, and Chiclet teeth.

Some ten million strong, the television audience's fascination with *The Swan*'s chronicle of the outer and supposed inner transformation of the contestants was matched by the disdain of the critics who lambasted everything from the New Age platitudes on transformation; the producers' exploitation of the participants for entertainment; the participants' willingness to be guinea pigs and sideshow attractions; the uniform aesthetic, which replaced whatever was unique and individual about each woman; the irresponsible and misleading presentation of numerous invasive procedures; and the underlying assumption that, for these women at least, looks were everything. Yet despite these criticisms, the show was a huge popular success. Were people drawn by, as one critic suggested, "that voyeuristic tendency to peek through the fingers of one hand while holding their noses with the other"?[9] Did the show's attraction rest on how easy it was for the viewer to feel good about herself, watching these women who were only in pursuit of physical changes they were too lazy and unmotivated to seek for themselves? Or did the background stories of the contestants—hard luck, bad luck, or no luck—simply make the viewer's life seem, by comparison, positively hunky dory? The combination of the hard luck story with a prize at the end was an old theme in television, one writer pointed out, linking 1950s shows like *Queen for a Day*, in which a contestant won a new appliance, with *The Swan*, where the prize was a new face.[10] Another critic suggested that while "cruelty has always made for good television," the fascination with *The Swan* was more a reflection of the viewer's own concern with being fat or out of shape.[11]

The shows became news, the participants minor celebrities, and numerous magazine and even newspaper articles focused on the aftershow follow-ups, asking the central question: Had these women really been transformed inside and out? Had a new nose, breasts, and sparkling smile done the trick? Were the contestants really better off?

Not altogether surprisingly, most of the stories denigrated both the contestants and their motives. One such story focused on Melissa Jones, formerly a "mousy, bespectacled outcast with protruding ears, a boxy nose, and flat chest" who had nonetheless dreamt of becoming a model. She underwent some $72,000 worth of procedures, which in Jones's eyes permitted her to "finally be myself." Lest the reader lose sight of what constituted a fulfilled self, the piece ended with Melissa Jones's own summation of the process, a statement that confirmed the worst about the show and served as a blanket indictment of the underlying motivation for seeking out cosmetic surgery in the first place: "I would have been a mute," she says, "just as long as I could be pretty."[12]

Depending on the point of view, the dialogue pertaining to cosmetic surgery had either risen to new heights or sunk to new depths. Even *People* magazine ran a story asking whether plastic surgery was "essential" or "barbaric and out of control."[13] Movie and television actresses—the very people who had helped by example to bring cosmetic surgery into the mainstream in the first place—were asked to weigh in. Even with the particular rigors and demands of their profession—its insistence that they remain unrealistically young and beautiful—their answers reflected the ambivalence with which our society views cosmetic surgery with answers that ranged from "yes" to "no" to "never." Forty-three-year-old actress Julianne Moore volunteered that "what I don't want is for people to stop looking like people or for there to be a homogenized sense of what's beautiful. I guess if I didn't feel it was an epidemic, I'd feel better about it."

The actress wasn't alone in thinking that the trend reflected aspects of contemporary culture in a harsh and unflattering light. All of the women on the reality shows ended up looking pretty much the same, suggesting that in a country obsessed with "follow-me consumerism," we might all end up with the same face or body, inspired by a celebrity or a trend.

In truth, this is an old theme, one famously portrayed in a *Twilight Zone* episode, "The Eye of the Beholder," first aired in November of 1960, and commented on in nearly every serious book about plastic surgery.

We watch as a young woman swathed in bandages pleads with her doctor to help her, saying, "I never wanted to be beautiful. I just wanted people not to scream when they looked at me." It is the last of eleven procedures, we learn, and if it fails, Miss Janet Tyler will be sent into exile with others like her. While the story is filtered through a contemporary Cold War lens (it is the Leader of the State who has decreed "glorious conformity"), it nonetheless delineates America's distrust of what was then still a fledgling practice limited to movie stars and the very privileged. In the end, the patient is revealed as blond and beautiful, while the doctors and nurses—who gasp when her face is shown at last—are all hideously pig-faced. The voice of Rod Serling makes the meaning crystalline: "Now the question comes to mind . . . where is this place and when is it, what kind of world where ugliness is the norm and beauty the deviation from the norm?" The answer is the Twilight Zone, of course.

In November of 2004, forty years later, *W* magazine—a periodical devoted to fashion, beauty, and celebrity, after all—asked a variation on the question in a piece entitled "The New Normal," which examined the concerns of some doctors who wondered "whether they are ushering in an age of bionic beauty, an era in which 'the new normal' is a cosmetically enhanced face or body." One doctor wondered out loud what the new standard of beauty would do to those who didn't choose surgery—would naturally beautiful women be considered ugly? The writer noted that since "in America, what's good for the celebrity gooses is automatically lusted after by the public gander," more "civilians" were seeking out extreme makeovers. The larger question, though, remained whether all of these trends signaled a fundamental change, a new vision of the physical self as a mere "shell" or "epidermal clothes which can be bought, new or used, and discarded when they fray or go out of style."[14]

The concerns voiced in the popular press had been raised earlier by members of the scholarly community at the Hastings Center for Ethics. Among the questions raised were those of professional ethics and the responsibility of the surgeon performing the enhancement. Philosopher Margaret Olivia Little asserted that what she called "cultural complicity" was at work in American society since standards of beauty—the preference for large breasts or small noses—were nothing more than social constructs. Little argued that while cosmetic surgery seemed to offer hope for individuals who felt that they fell outside of those standards of beauty—because they were flat-chested or had big noses—the rising number of breast augmentations and rhinoplasties performed by doctors simply entrenched those standards more deeply. These standards, she insisted, were, in fact, "suspect" norms of appearance.[15]

She was not alone in seeing the trends in cosmetic surgery as reflecting a raft of social ills. Conservative writer Christine Rosen called cosmetic surgery "a useful Fathometer for assessing the state of our democracy and a Rorschach test for people's views about much broader social currents: the glorification of youth, the tenor of popular culture, the peculiar but strenuous American anxiety about identity." She argued that our society has come to see plastic surgery as an answer to the inequalities built into a culture where "beauty is a valuable commodity that is unfairly distributed," and declared that the culture's solution was "to democratize beauty, to make it something that, fueled by envy and with enough money and effort, anyone can attain." Rosen viewed our embrace of cosmetic surgery as embodying "potential harms—both to individuals and to society as a whole," supplanting "moral education" with superficial, external markers of health, beauty, and success.[16]

The moral basis for Rosen's carefully parsed argument is moored in contemporary trends, but when she wrote that "we are not yet a nation of Narcissi, content to stare happily into the pool, our surgically enhanced self-esteem intact but our character irrevocably compromised," her words reflect two older currents in American thought. The first assumes that changes wrought by surgery are only superficial in nature and also morally suspect as well as inimical to "a life-long process of moral education."[17] The second theme—overcoming "nature"—is one inextricably bound up with both religious thinking as well as a distrust of medicine and technology as trespassing into areas that belong rightly to God, not man.

We are taught from the very first that anything good or desirable is worth working for. In the same way that we esteem money earned over inherited wealth, we value physical transformation when it involves diet (discipline) and exercise (work). Physical transformation achieved by other means—by liposuction, for example—neither reflects on the individual's achievement, since it doesn't require discipline or work, nor is it intrinsically valuable. The relative ease with which cosmetic surgery achieves its results isn't to be trusted, the Puritan strain in our society tells us; the individual willing to choose this "easy" way out must do so out of a flaw or an unhealthy impulse because, as a group, we distrust the "quick fix." Even Elizabeth Haiken, whose book is a thorough and relatively dispassionate history of cosmetic surgery, notes that while cosmetic surgery seems to reflect the American dream's "promise of individual transformation," nonetheless it "subverts our most cherished hopes even as it seems to fulfill them." She writes that cosmetic surgery is both "a cause and a consequence of a loss of faith in the possibility of transformation on a broader scale."[18] Haiken's view accurately captures not only our distrust of the physical transformation cosmetic surgery offers, but our suspicion that it actually impedes true, inner transformation.

These ideas about true transformation draw on other, older themes, among them the skin as the mere outer envelope of the self and, therefore, cosmetic surgery as the most "shallow" (in all senses) of surgery. When surgery involves other parts of the body—when it goes "inside," the locus we identify with the self—we are ready to believe that inner transformation and surgery can and do go hand in hand, as many magazine articles and books attest. The former drinker with a liver transplant, the ex-smoker with a new heart, the overweight and unexercised man with a triple bypass, and even the reformed overeater with a stapled stomach are understood as believable living testaments to the combined power of surgery and the "second chance" to effect internal, spiritual change. Diet, exercise, and denial of appetite and impulse are seen as disciplines when viewed through this lens—exertions of the inner self on the outer body, as well as demonstrations of self-control, self-determination, and self-realization.

Cosmetic surgery, which appears to deal with only the surface and, most important, is wrought by a third party, doesn't make the grade. But since all surgery is, by its very nature, performed by a third party, we have to assume that it is the "surface" on which cosmetic surgery is performed that makes the difference.

Most important, our ideas about the self and selfhood locate the essence of who we are on the inside. Our Western perspective incorporates Greek philosophy, Judeo-Christian ideas, as well as the Cartesian divide; we talk about "mind," "spirit," or "soul" as wholly separate from the body. As Susan Bordo notes, in Western culture, the soul and the body are not only separate, but at odds. The body is "animal" and the place of fleshly "appetites" in contrast to the higher spirit and soul; the body belongs to earth while the soul connects to heaven. The body has also been viewed historically as "the prison of the soul and confounder of its projects." Most important, she writes that "what remains the constant through historical variation is the *construction* of body as something apart from the true self (whether conceived as soul, mind, spirit, will, creativity, freedom . . .) and as undermining the best efforts of that self."[19]

As a result, as members of our culture, we harbor more than a sneaking suspicion that paying too much attention to the surface—the things that are "only" skin-deep—may actually be detrimental to the health of the soul. This formulation becomes pivotal when it comes to our cultural assessment of women who choose cosmetic surgery.

Just as we value that which is hard-earned over that which is acquired with ease, we value beauty that is "natural" over beauty that is enhanced for both aesthetic and moral reasons. We hang on to the belief that natural is better (and more valuable); we prefer the "real" redhead or blonde, the "born" beauty, despite the fact that images of beauty have been idealized for thousands of years, long before digital or surgical enhancement. The impulse to adorn or improve our appearance certainly is as old as the race itself, though the standard of what constitutes beauty (plump or thin, big-breasted or small, curly-haired or straight, and the like) changes decade by decade, century by century, even within a single society. None of that changes our stubborn, if not always articulated, conviction that "real" or "natural" is always better. Parenthetically, that conviction also keeps the covers of magazines devoted to celebrities preoccupied with stories about which star has been surgically enhanced.

And then there is the potent theme of the limits of technology—that point on the human grid where what we *can* do medically and technologically intersects with the question of what we *should* do. In the twenty-first century, the need to answer the question seems even more urgent as medical advances rapidly increase what we can do. But the way in which we frame the question of what we should do remains informed and shaped by much older ways of thinking.

How deeply entrenched these older ideas are in American culture is demonstrated by a story called "The Birthmark," written by Nathaniel Hawthorne in 1846. Its story line needs to be only slightly updated to make it a contemporary parable about the limits of science and the dangers of society's pursuit of physical perfection. These themes underlie many of the objections to cosmetic surgery and other medical technologies today.

Aylmer, a scientist who has devoted his life to seeking out "man's ultimate control of nature," leaves his laboratory long enough to fall in love with and marry a beautiful young woman named Georgiana. She is exquisite, save for a curious birthmark on her cheek, formed in the shape of a hand. After their marriage, Aylmer becomes increasingly obsessed with the birthmark, and finally confronts his wife, saying, "You came so nearly perfect from the hand of Nature that this slightest possible defect, which we hesitate to term a defect or a beauty, shocks me as being the visible mark of earthly imperfection." Even though he tries to be tactful—hedging on whether the mark is a thing of beauty or a defect—what he truly feels is painfully clear to his wife. Georgiana is both hurt and surprised by his obsession, partly because, as we learn, men attracted to her had always thought the birthmark proof of her "magic endowments," perhaps placed by a "fairy's hand." While her female rivals gloated that the discoloration marred her beauty, men were charmed by it. Aylmer, though, can only see it as an emblem of "the fatal flaw of humanity."

Georgiana, made miserable by Aylmer's alienation, agrees to

have him try to remove it. After several abortive experiments, Aylmer concocts a potion that brings a wilted and dying plant back to life, thus restoring it to perfection. He then applies the formula to his wife's cheek. But, as the birthmark fades and then disappears, Georgiana begins to lose consciousness and, in the end, dies. Hawthorne leaves the moral eminently clear, writing that Aylmer had "grappled with the mystery of life" and had failed, as a human being, to "find the perfect future in the present."

In addition to the main theme of man's tampering with nature (and, by extension, God's creation), Hawthorne also explores the connection between identity and appearance. Aylmer cannot see Georgiana for who she is—a woman of fulsome humanity, filled with love, generosity, and kindness—because of the birthmark. What Aylmer sees as imperfection is, at the same time, the symbol of all that constitutes both her identity and her humanity. In the most profound of senses, the birthmark is who she is, and by destroying it, Aylmer destroys her. The suspicion, if not the conviction, that changing our appearances by technological means (such as cosmetic surgery) must involve a loss of identity and that the pursuit of such perfection is, in and of itself, morally deleterious remains a potent and persistent thread in American thought.

While the debate about the proper limits of scientific or technological intervention is centuries old—Mary Shelley's *Frankenstein* was published in 1817—for some critics, the incredible scientific and medical progress achieved in the last fifty years has made the debate all the more urgent. Cosmetic surgery is at the heart of this debate for reasons both historical and contemporary.

In his book, *Better than Well: American Medicine Meets the American Dream*, Carl Elliott argues that focusing on self-improvement as what is morally important about enhancement technologies is "unhelpful and misleading." Instead, he puts his finger on what he considers America's moral dilemma: "The question is not whether there is any moral cost to the quest to become *better* but whether there is any moral cost to the quest to become *different*." Sweeping in all the enhancements our consumer society offers—from accent reduction clinics to cosmetic surgery to drugs, such as Prozac, which can change us in other ways—he writes, "If we have mixed feelings [about these technologies], it is partly because we have mixed feelings about the visions of the good life these technologies serve."[20]

Nathaniel Hawthorne would have understood the argument well.

The War Against Women: The Feminist Position

Since the preponderance of cosmetic procedures are performed on women by men, the question of agency occupies the heart of the feminist arguments against cosmetic surgery. This has been true since the 1991 publication of Naomi Wolf's best-selling and influential book *The Beauty Myth*, which, ironically, coincided with the exponential rise in cosmetic surgeries. In fact, a year later, the Association of Plastic Surgeons began for the first time to track both the number and types of surgeries performed by its members.

Wolf's parsing of cosmetic surgery—discussed in a chapter titled "Violence"—was unflinchingly antagonistic, and attributed women's willingness to undergo surgery to the inability to break from a history of male oppression. Central to her argument was the fact that not only were the preponderance of cosmetic surgeons men but that the "violence" of cosmetic surgery was inherently political. Wolf understood cosmetic surgery as part of an assault on the embodied female, for "whatever is deeply essentially female—the life in a woman's expression, the feel of her flesh, the shape of her breasts, the transformations after childbirth of her skin—is being reclassified as ugly, and ugliness as disease."[21] Rather than deriding women's choices to undergo surgery as narcissistic, Wolf instead suggested that the desperation for beauty came from another source, holding "on to a sexual center" that was threatened both by the ageism in our society and our culture's demand that women be physically perfect. Finally, Wolf concluded that along with the threat of "lost love comes the threat of invisibility," and that "women have face-lifts in a society in which women without them vanish from sight."[22]

Wolf's passion was in part inspired by what she rightly saw well over a decade ago as the trivialization of surgical procedures, something she witnessed firsthand growing up in New York City. She noted with not a little irony that even the popular terms by which surgical procedures are known revealed cultural manipulation: "Cosmetic surgery is not 'cosmetic,' and human flesh is not 'plastic.' Trivialization and infantilization pervade the surgeons' language when they speak to women: 'a nip,' a 'tummy tuck . . .' This baby talk falsifies reality. Surgery changes one forever, the mind as well as the body."[23]

Wolf's point of view has been echoed by other writers, among them Susan Bordo in an essay countering Kathy Davis's assertion in *Shaping the Female Body* that women who chose surgery acted out of a sense of agency. Bordo asserts that escaping the pressure of our culture—a culture in which "the surgically perfect body . . . has become the model of the 'normal' "—is well-nigh impossible, as the "ante" of "what counts as an acceptable face and body" is continually "upped." Further, she writes that "in focusing on the narratives of individual 'empowerment,' Davis—like Oprah's guests who claim they did it 'for themselves'—overlooks the fact that the norms that encourage these individuals to see themselves as defective are enmeshed in the practice and institution of cosmetic surgery itself. And so is individual behavior."[24]

But this way of thinking suggests that all the women who come into my office or any other to choose surgery—and I am one of them—are casualties of low self-esteem or insecurity and unwitting victims of a female-hating culture, rather than adults choosing freely and acting autonomously. Do we really believe that breasts and faces are *always* lifted, eyes done, thighs slimmed not for the self but for pleasing the "other," whether we identify that other as a lover or hus-band, the demands of a career, or the standards of beauty imposed by society at large? I would be quick to admit that some women choose surgery solely for those reasons (I try to weed these women out of my practice, since I have discovered that surgery will prove less than sat-isfying for them), but *all* of them? Do we really believe that women are incapable of choosing for themselves, by themselves?

There are, after all, other pressures imposed on women by our culture, beyond a "perfect" body or face. There is undeniable pressure to marry, for example, and to have children, and yet we never think of women who marry or who become mothers as lacking in agency or as cultural victims. Nor do we see women who don't marry or don't have children as necessarily stronger, truer, more independent than women who do. Why should we accept other narratives of choice or "empowerment"—whether published as nonfiction or heard at din-ner from a friend—as authentic and sometimes uplifting, but suspect those pertaining to cosmetic surgery? We will take the woman at her word who tells us why she became a lawyer or a doctor, or why she left her husband, but not the woman who decided she wanted a facelift or a nose job for reasons she considered valid and important. Why do we insist that women who choose to have cosmetic surgery aren't really choosing for themselves, but are always being manipu-lated by cultural norms?

My patients and their behavior illuminate the process of agency and choice. I show them books filled with photographs of fresh, red scars, and watch their faces as they take in the details of the sur-gery they are contemplating. There is little sugarcoating in my office about what surgery entails. While there are techniques in certain sur-geries to make the scars less visible, I insist that the patient know and understand that there is no such thing as scarless surgery—despite what those pop-up ads on the computer desktop or in the backs of magazines may promise—and I pay attention as she takes in the information and permits it to inform her conscious choice. Breast reduction, for example, will leave significant scarring and may involve loss of nipple sensation—a trade-off the patient must consider.

Anxiety—beginning anywhere from a few weeks to a few hours before surgery—is a normal reaction and is usually focused on the fear associated with anesthesia. The anxiety may be minimal—most patients find themselves very busy before an operation—but it is almost always reflected in repeated phone calls and questions to the office right before the surgery. Although there is certainly a fair amount of protective denial in people who are facing surgery, whether it is elective or not, very few patients actually believe surgery is entirely free of risk. And then there is recovery—a very different process from what the so-called "weekend" facelifts advertised in magazines suggest. After surgery, the patient wakes up in the operating or recovery room. The staff—the nurses and anesthesiologist—orient her back into the world with words such as: "You are awakening from surgery. It is Thursday, two P.M. You are okay, and everything went well."

Recovery is a vulnerable and humbling period, since most patients will experience a combination of pain and helplessness. Old traumas may reemerge, and needs may be felt more intensely. Many patients have drains that collect blood and fluid from the wound after the surgery—a detail that gives the invasive nature of the surgery a graphic reality—and while each patient must decide on her own how to cope with this aspect of recovery, choose she must. There is usually real discomfort and pain associated with recuperation. Blood on the sheets and bandages are part of the undeniable evidence of a wound and, later, a scar.

If the willingness to take on all these aspects of surgery doesn't entail agency, I would ask, What does?

And yet, without apology, the contemporary view of women who undertake cosmetic surgery as malleable and easily herded into unhealthy decisions, the targeted and hapless consumers of medical enhancement, prevails, as Sheila M. Rothman and David J. Rothman write in *The Pursuit of Perfection: The Promise and Perils of Medi-*

cal Enhancement.[25] To go along with this view, I would have to ignore all the stories I have heard from women over the years pertaining to the choice to undergo surgery. Most important, I would have to discount the personal narratives told to me by patients who have undergone surgery in the face of illness and accident and have returned to elect cosmetic surgery for themselves. Each of these narratives, in its own way, illuminates how elective surgery can be a tool of literal and symbolic transformation. The following story is a variant on a larger theme, since a significant percentage of my breast reconstruction patients later return for elective surgery.

Susan was a beautiful young woman in her early twenties whose uneven gait and shoulders testified to the severe spinal deformities she had been born with. As a child, she'd undergone seven or eight operations to correct her birth defects—all of which she recalled as painful, traumatic, and highly disruptive to all the activities we normally associate with childhood. And yet she was in my office to discuss elective surgery—breast augmentation. Her breasts were very small and somewhat asymmetrical, which might have been a result of all of her previous surgeries. I asked her the same question I ask all my patients: "Why now?"

She answered me in a clear voice, unhesitating, as her mother listened, seated by her side. She'd graduated from college and was looking forward to starting her first job in another city. She was, as she put it, "moving on," and she wanted to mark the beginning of what she called her "own life" and the end of her childhood. She wanted this for herself because she felt it would make her feel sexier and more feminine, on the one hand, and truly "launched" and independent on the other. She had chosen this for herself and it was clear that her mother was there only for support. I understood that she saw the breast augmentation as an act of self-assertion, an undertaking very different in kind from the many surgeries she'd had to submit to as a child. Even when I explained the risks of the procedure—the scarring, the lifetime maintenance of the implants—she was undeterred. She wanted this for herself and she saw it as a way of marking the new path opening for her in life.

Despite the lens through which our culture views cosmetic surgery, as a display of weakness or insecurity, choosing to change the body through surgery and assume its risks can indeed be both an assertion of the self and a vehicle for self-transformation.

Rethinking the Mind-Body Split

All of the cultural arguments against cosmetic surgery—and the subsequent shame or embarrassment women may feel after electing to have it—rely on the assumption that the "mind" or the soul is superior to the "body" and that the two share no relationship other than, perhaps, an antagonistic one. Importantly, this assumption isn't based on what science now knows about the mind-body connection in the twenty-first century, which, in the West, is only now being examined in depth. Despite what our culture asserts, the body is much more than an exterior surface and is intimately connected to the self and its development. Researchers acknowledge that work on the mind-body connection is still in its infancy, and our understanding of how the mind and the body connect to create the entity we call the self still needs to be filled out in detail.

Still, science has recognized that the experiences of the body always shape the mind as well and that the mind, in both sickness and health, can work to change and shape the body. The mind-body split, which has been a cornerstone of Western thought for centuries, has ceased to serve us, both as individuals and as a culture. More specifically, it is the foundation for our ambivalence about cosmetic surgery as well as the source of our confusion about how healing the body and the mind takes place.

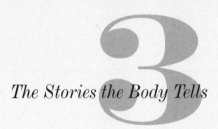

The Stories the Body Tells

The presumption of the mind-body split is woven into both the fabric of our culture and the way our culture trains its surgeons. Part of my journey has, of necessity, included unlearning the physical and emotional detachment my medical training engrained in me so that my "mind" would be my primary resource as a physician. I've had to revise my view of the mind-body relationship taught by the Western medical establishment. And, as a woman in a field dominated by men, I have also had to reclaim my feminine body and learn to listen to it. In the process, I have grown in understanding, and I believe I have become a better listener as well as a better doctor.

I ended up in medical school after taking "the road less traveled"—I was an English major and fine arts minor in college and spent several years before and after college studying art in formal settings. But there was a part of me—practical, no doubt—that couldn't quite envision the instability of the artist's life. I was also drawn to new therapies that emphasized the connections among body, mind, and spirit, and that weren't part of the Western model of healing; I was certified in biofeedback and studied several other "alternative" therapies. Finally, I thought that the grounding in medical science—

missing from all the various therapies I had studied that focused on a part of the whole—would allow me to see beyond the limitations of each specialized approach to healing.

My own plans for my future in medicine were admittedly vague: A country doctor, perhaps, or a psychiatrist, healing families and children? I didn't know precisely, but I was in search of a kind of doctoring that would bring body and soul together. As it happens, I got to medical school precisely at the moment when specialization was the model for medicine, particularly at Stanford—no more Dr. Welby, general practitioner—and for some years, I cast about, quite miserably, for a niche that I could find truly satisfying. Psychiatry turned out to be less about dream work, Freud, and Jung—the part the humanist and mystic in me loved—than about drugs and neurobiology, and I clocked many hours as a medical student researching sleep patterns and slicing up rats' brains to investigate neural pathways. I began to realize that the kind of questions I liked to ask—"Can the brain understand the mind?" "Where is the seat of the soul?" "What constitutes physical reality?"—weren't part of the protocol of the lab setting and didn't seem to endear me to my colleagues. To put it kindly, I didn't fit in precisely.

Cardiac surgery at Stanford was exciting and cutting-edge—heart transplants, dramatic life-or-death moments, helicopter rides, and handsome surgeons in cowboy boots—but the specialty was pretty much male terrain, and I had the wisdom to notice that the one formerly brunette female resident in the department had actually gone gray in a single year. Self-preservation prevailed, leaving me once again in search of the specialty of my dreams.

In the end, I turned to plastic surgery. At first it seemed a counterintuitive choice—how could removing or altering a part heal the whole?—but Stanford's training emphasized reconstruction and focused on birth defects, burns, and severe injuries. I thought the surgery I was being trained to do was necessary, and the healing it offered evident.

Virtually nothing about surgical training was about wholeness or healing. While women are a more significant presence in medical schools all over the country today, it wasn't true then, some twenty-five years ago, and the initiation into what one anthropologist has called the "martial, masculine ambiance of surgery" wasn't without its hardships.[1] (It's worth remembering that while 87 percent of plastic surgery patients are female, as of 2004, only 6 percent of board-certified surgeons were women.)

The dispassion—or the emotional disconnect—required to look at grievous injury or to cut into living flesh isn't something that came to me naturally. I remember the first time I went on rounds and confronted my first infected abdominal wound—the sight and sickly sweet smell of exposed intestines—and immediately registered the shock by turning green and excusing myself to the bathroom, much to the chief resident's displeasure. Curt and to the point, he dressed me down, and told me to go home if I couldn't take it. He didn't leave it at that: He said he didn't want me "infecting" him or the others with the "sickness" I had. In the context of surgical training, my first reaction, completely understandable and certainly human, became a sign of weakness, of metaphorical "infection," perhaps even of "femaleness," since I was one of the first all-female groups of residents. I left in tears and returned the next morning as a person with a shell around my heart. I tried not to show any sign of vulnerability after that—which, I suppose, in the surgical-training scheme of things, "proved" that the chief resident's tactic had been a rousing success. I would end up crying only once in public during the remaining seven years of my training.

The "martial, masculine ambiance" of surgical training had another cost. I felt keenly that each year of my training—thirteen years in all—pushed me further away from my true gifs of intuition and compassion as a healer. Those qualities didn't fit into the model of surgery; I became, as I was supposed to, tough and decisive, and used my brain over my heart in every situation. In retrospect, it was a process that gradually weaned me away from my feminine strengths—among them, intuitive knowledge and empathy—qualities that I would later need to reclaim myself. Becoming attached to a patient in this context was a sign of weakness, as was being horrified at the way patients were depersonalized. My sense of self was challenged by the training in small ways and large; the women in the program were to banish all things that might be considered part of our female identity in the pursuit of surgical excellence. No mascara (they maintained it could flake into the wound) and no earrings (they could fall off) were among the many other "nos." Even my ankle bracelet was deemed unprofessional, not surprisingly when that super-male model of the surgeon was all there was. And yet even with every cultural mark of "femininity" removed, not even the unisex uniform of the blue scrubs we all wore could disguise the fact I was what anthropologist Joan Cassell has called "a woman in a surgeon's body."

Political correctness stops us from talking about the body in this way—or about the possible differences between men and women as surgeons—but the connections between the body, surgery, and the surgeon are profound and complex.

Among the medical specialties, surgery is uniquely embodied and physical because, as Joan Cassell comments, "surgeries involve bodies—those of the surgeons as well as the patients. During an operation, the body of the surgeon makes brutal contact with the body of the patient, piercing the envelope of the skin, assaulting the flesh, violating bodily integrity."[2] But I knew intuitively that the contact between the surgeon's body and that of the patient wasn't as "brutal" or depersonalized as my training made it seem. I felt that plastic surgery, like art, is loving creation. Today I would say categorically that surgery is the most physically intimate contact two consenting adults can have other than sex.

Surgery is embodied in another sense, in that the surgeon's body is part of the process since he or she relies on his or her senses of sight, sound, touch, and smell. Surgery is indeed "hands-on" as well as intuitive; later, when I taught residents at Stanford, the hardest part was explaining those aspects of surgery—the judgments and actions—that are intuitively based. You learn to operate by practicing; these are skills mastered by doing and absorbing—like performing a plié or catching a football—not by thinking or talking. Yet for all that the practice of surgery depends on the surgeon's body in these ways, what has been called the "ethos" of surgical training forcibly disconnects the trainee from his or her body in ways that are both real and metaphorical. I learned to ignore what my body was telling me—whether I was hungry or tired or ill. All of those attitudes are literally "incorporated" into the surgeon-in-training's own body.

The extreme sleep deprivation of residency has been described before in other places, but that doesn't detract from the experience of it. It is, in every sense, unbelievable. I cried for the second and last time one night when I covered the emergency room while the chief resident slept. I'd been up for a full twenty-four hours. There were forty or so people on the neurosurgery floor under my care, and in the wee hours of the night, more admissions rolled in. A drunken man cursed at me while I sutured a large cut on his face. A severely burned child was in need of help. There were people on gurneys in the emergency room hallways. The tipping point came when a woman with self-inflicted lacerations to her arms and legs came in and I did what every senior resident knew *never* to do: I called and woke up the chief resident, then asked him to come and help me. Calling him may have been born of desperation, but given the setting, it also took enormous guts on my part. He was predictably angry. He looked at the lacerations and immediately ordered a staple gun. To my horror, he started stapling the lacerations without anesthesia and then handed me the gun to finish. Dazed, I melted down. I sat at the nursing station, put my head into my hands, and cried. No one said a word, probably because no one knew what to say. After what seemed like an eternity, an older nurse came up behind me and patted me on the shoulder. It was a welcome reminder that there was still some warmth left in the world.

There were other ways I felt disenfranchised. As a woman, I was outside the circle of male surgeons and outside the circle of the other women—the nurses—who made up the small world of the hospital. There were the flirtations and sexual intrigues primarily between the male doctors and female nurses that have made hospitals a prime setting for television dramas. I remember sleeping in the cardiac resident's call room one night when someone knocked on the door at two A.M. I opened the door to find a nurse, a bottle of wine tucked under her arm. We were, as I recall, equally surprised by the encounter.

Looking back, I see my own struggle to maintain the female self in the surgical scrubs more clearly than I even saw it then. I know that I felt my feminine "self" under assault, which I experienced, not surprisingly, in an embodied way. And it was in that context that I sought to reclaim myself through my body by choosing to alter it. I had my first cosmetic surgery—a rhinoplasty to smooth out the bump in my nose and open up my airway passages—during my third year of residency. While my operation certainly helped me breathe more easily, both literally and metaphorically, it had other more profound effects.

It's no accident that the nose I had altered was my father's ethnic and genetic legacy to me, and that by changing it, I was signaling my independence from him and his expectations. Then, too, at a time when I felt myself becoming more and more "masculine"—less capable of feminine "softness"—altering the most masculine of my features was a re-assertion of that feminine self. By having surgery, I felt I was reclaiming my woman's face—the most public part of the physical self—in a real and specific way. Because I did not want my colleagues to know—I knew they would see my surgery as a sign of weakness or insecurity—I insisted that the surgeon leave the bones intact. My recovery was quick and the physical change in my nose slight—barely visible from the front, slightly more pronounced in profile. But the change inside me was more profound than the reflection of my smoothed-out nose in the mirror. I felt transformed by the surgery, which announced both a renewed and new "me"; ironically, the only regret I've ever had is that I didn't allow the surgeon to go a bit further and make my nose just a bit smaller and softer. It's probably not a coincidence that I met the man I would soon marry right after the surgery.

My own surgery certainly provided me with a personal glimpse at the connection between the outside self and the inner one, but even so, at the time I hadn't an inkling how complicated the relationship is. The myriad connections between the "self"—that entity we know exists but cannot find a single physical location for—and the body which is its physical manifestation began to reveal themselves as I came into contact with more patients and as my work began to move into territories more complicated than the terra firma of reconstructive surgery.

Written on the Body

One day, on surgical rotation in a busy hospital, I rushed into a room where an adolescent boy sat on the patient's table, with his mother by his side. It was a clinic where a two- or three-hour wait was the norm and the doctors more or less sprinted from one room to another. The boy's hair was cut very short, highlighting the fact that his ears stood at right angles to his head. Filled with more than a little overconfidence, I greeted them with the words, "So, you've come to have your ears pinned back? We can definitely help you with that!" The smile still on my face, I turned to the mother, whose face had turned to stone as she put a protective arm around her son. Her voice rising with anger, she informed me that there was *nothing* wrong with her boy's ears. They were, in fact, in the clinic to consult about a bump on his nose.

To my eye—and probably everyone else's—the "bump" was practically invisible; his ears, on the other hand, were another story. But I still wasn't understanding that place of connection between "self" and "perception." It was a difficult meeting but I learned that both the boy's father and grandfather had the same ears and that he had been brought up to see his ears not simply as endearing but as part of his connection to his family and its legacy. In his personal context, how his ears looked had taken on a very different meaning from the norm society imposed. The bump was another matter entirely and they wanted that bump gone.

The dressing-down I received from the chief of surgery, to whom the mother complained, only underscored the first important lesson I had learned as a plastic surgeon who'd ventured beyond the realm of "reconstruction."

It was the last time I would ever walk into an examining room with a preconceived idea of why a patient was there. My first question now is *always* "Why have you come to see me?" because what I see may bear no relationship to what the patient sees when he or she looks in the mirror. I became a better listener and, by listening, began to understand about the roles "perception" and "story" play in the individual's attitude toward his or her body as a whole, as well as its parts. The boy's ears were "storied" in the sense that they had been given an important and meaningful context that effectively turned on its head the idea that they were a "defect". Even though I have no way of knowing what happened to the boy from all those years ago whose mother taught me an important lesson, I think about him now and then. He would be a man by now and I sometimes wonder if his family's "story" about his ears survived the years of his adolescence and early adulthood. Did teasing in high school or a remark by someone he admired help to supplant his family's "story" with another "story" from the outside world? If it did, he might well have found himself walking into another plastic surgeon's office one day, asking to have his ears pinned back.

I soon understood that the young man's case was the rule, not the exception. Each and every one of us has positive and negative meanings and stories attached to our bodies, beginning, research has suggested, as early as infancy. Some of the first stories are set in place during our childhood when shared familial traits are often commented upon; from the time I was small, I knew that "having" my father's nose, curly hair, and big feet in the context of my family's stories meant more than simply sharing physical characteristics. While we're growing up, the stories we incorporate about our bodies are reflections not only of contemporary social constructs pertaining to beauty and attractiveness but of the views and opinions of the closer society of friends and family as well as ourselves. We endow our bodies with personal mythology, which is both a part of our story of the self and, at the same time, shapes the self's story.

Our linguistic expressions have long acknowledged this other aspect of embodiment even before science examined and proved it, showing that we each see not just ourselves but others in both literal and symbolic or storied ways. We may comment that someone's "honesty shows in her face" or that someone "radiates calm" or that "the eyes are the window to the soul." We don't mean this literally, of course; we are actually describing the inner self as we imagine it to be reflected in the body. Drawing from our own personal experience—the large hands of a beloved uncle or the round cheeks of a doting grandmother—we may endow with meaning certain physical characteristics in others.

Research has confirmed what I observed in my practice, showing that body image is, in fact, almost wholly "storied" in this sense and has surprisingly little to do with the "objective" reality of how we actually look. This finding will be familiar to most of us who have experienced bewilderment or surprise—and then shock or pleasure—when we see ourselves in photographs or videos or on television, or when we look at an old photo from a time we felt positively fat and see a nicely proportioned or even thin young woman. Research confirms that there is little overlap between subjective body image (that is, what the person sees from the "inside") and measures of objective attractiveness (what the "outside" world sees and evaluates). Basically this means that a beautiful appearance validated by society doesn't guarantee a positive body image and, conversely, a more ordinary appearance doesn't always result in a negative one.[3] Parenthetically, it explains why some famously beautiful women are often prone to confess that, despite all the adulation they receive, they do not "feel" beautiful. Body image evolves over the life span and is more dimensional than the simple act of looking in a mirror would suggest. It's been proposed that physical characteristics are only one of four components that make up an individual's body image. "Cultural socialization"—all the standards and expectations society communicates about appearance—is another. This is vast territory in our media-saturated culture and one that, research shows, affects small children, adolescents, and adults.

But body image is also affected by personal experience—everything the individual has heard about his or her appearance from family, friends, and even strangers. These experiences can be positive and validating—as in the boy's "story" about his ears—or negative and destructive to the sense of self. Cultural socialization and personal experiences provide the context for personal narratives about the body, which are shaped by physical characteristics and personality factors.

Personality factors affect both how we evaluate what we see in the mirror and how we absorb what we've learned from the culture and the people closest to us. We've all had firsthand experience of how this works with the gorgeous girlfriend who is always focused on her flaws and is never satisfied with her looks. Or we might have known the amazingly self-confident girl who, even though she wasn't conventionally attractive, attracted more attention than the conventionally beautiful one because she really knew how to strut her stuff. High self-esteem can protect the individual against negative outside influences while low self-esteem can make her more vulnerable to them. Women and girls who are perfectionists are less buffered than those who are not. Body image is, in fact, slippery and complicated terrain.

But "body image"—despite what it sounds like—isn't only about appearance. The term is actually misleading since the word *image* suggests a mental representation or picture, but "body image"—which is what researchers call it for want of a better term—is far more complex and multidimensional. It's not just how we perceive our bodies but how we experience them. As Thomas Cash and Thomas Pruzinsky write, "Our most fundamental sense of ourselves is as a body. The sense of self is based on the experience that one is embodied and differentiated from the outside world."[4] While Descartes ventured that "I think, therefore I am," modern science's version might well be "I am because I have a body and am not you." Despite the cultural notion that the body is only the surface of the self, the body is intimately connected to the entity we call the self, since everything we experience is experienced through it. As David W. Krueger explains, "An idea as well as a fact, the body is a container and conduit of emotional experience, and the body image a Rorshach onto which fantasies, meaning, and significance are projected."[5] In addition, each individual endows parts of the body with powerful symbolism that goes beyond the symbolism supplied by cultural narratives. So, for example, while the breast may symbolize femininity and nurturance for an individual, that symbolism will be expanded and personalized by the individual's life experiences.

The body and the self, long thought to be separate, are indeed intimately connected.

Seeing the young boy that day swung open a door for me, and my day-to-day experiences made me realize again and again that the world I lived and worked in wasn't black and white. Even though all the work I was doing was technically "reconstructive" (and thus covered by health insurance), the gray areas were immediately clear. The definition of what was "necessary" to "reconstruct" expanded slightly over the years (and is now contracting rapidly)—sweeping in, over time, jug and cauliflower ears, uneven breasts, too-big breasts, and even, after much debate, reconstructing breasts surgically removed after cancer. As a resident, I had a firsthand look at how body image worked in a real-life setting. Private practice gave me an even closer look.

Within the storied nature of body image are the body parts with which women express satisfaction or dissatisfaction, and not surprisingly, they are "storied" as well. Encounters with patients proved this again and again as I learned that whatever "objective reality" cup size might reflect had nothing at all to do with how a woman "saw" her breasts. One woman's "too-large" breasts might be precisely what the next patient desired and, indeed, women come to my office in equal numbers for both augmentation and reduction. Perceptions of "fat" were equally storied and, in that sense, wholly personal; beautifully toned and extremely fit women will come into my office to consult about "fat" that would be virtually unnoticeable to a woman with a body less fit and toned. Elective surgery, it became clearer and clearer, had more to do with "story" than anything the mirror reflected.

My own personal experience with a second procedure taught me even more. While I initially chose to have liposuction to assert myself at a moment of life transition, its effects weren't as positive as my nose job had been and revealed the complexity of body image in another way, this time immediate and personal. It also taught me that, like body image, the "why" of electing surgery may sometimes be connected to "stories" we do not immediately recognize but which will determine whether we feel the surgery has been successful and the degree to which we have been transformed. It hinted that the connections between mind and body and their relation to healing were more specific and complicated than I had previously suspected.

I had my liposuction at thirty-five, after my residency and

divorce. I had dieted constantly during my marriage—there was great pressure on me to be "thin"—but I hated the way my breasts and curves simply disappeared when I got down to 125 pounds. But, inevitably, when I started to gain weight, not only would my breasts come back but so would the fat on my thighs and abdomen—a trait other women on my mother's side of the family have struggled with. Needless to say, these parts of my body were "storied" in the negative sense from earliest childhood when the other older women in the family complained about them incessantly. If my nose connected me to my father, where I tended to gain weight connected me to my mother. I thought a new cutting-edge technique would leave me with natural results and solve the problem of looking feminine without feeling "fat."

I did not heal in the ways I expected after the liposuction. It remains, to this day, the procedure I regret having. Ironically, the new body image it bequeathed me—some scarring and numbness and a new tendency to gain weight in my breasts, where it is very hard to lose—set me back rather than transformed me in a positive sense. Even though I meant to have the surgery as a celebration of my life as a newly single woman and a doctor forging her way alone in the world of private practice, it didn't take long for me to realize that I had done it primarily to look "thin." It was an act of self-criticism more than anything else. I had internalized both the general cultural ideals of what a woman's body should look like and the comments of others throughout my life. How I felt after the liposuction was in marked contrast to how I felt after my rhinoplasty, which had proved healing in every sense of the word.

The experience also convinced me that satisfaction with the results of cosmetic surgery might have little to do with what a woman sees in the mirror afterward, but might relate instead to whether she has come to terms with her own body's story. Perhaps women who aren't self-aware in this way and who were mainly influenced by the cultural norms would always end up both unchanged and mostly dissatisfied? Why was it that for some patients the change remained superficial while for others it entailed real transformation of the self? Did the surgery have to be preceded by self-knowledge for the patient to benefit in a real sense?

I started looking at my patients differently, and it soon became clear that some women who walked through my door were trying to please someone other than themselves. The women who came in with men who did all the talking. The pushy mothers with adolescent daughters in tow, some of them eager to please and others clearly rebellious. Women with photographs torn out of magazines who were yearning to be someone else. Women obsessed with how they looked. The women who thought that changing their physical selves would get them whatever eluded them in life—whether it was love, popularity, or money. These were all women who, in the end, wouldn't be satisfied with the results because they were looking for something cosmetic surgery couldn't give them: a validation of their own self-worth.

These are precisely the women I would learn to actively discourage from having surgery.

Over time, as I worked with my patients, it became clear that the stories of the body were always stories of the self.

Breast augmentation is one of the most frequently requested procedures in my office, as it is elsewhere in the United States. Though media coverage would have you believe that most women who elect this procedure are motivated to look like Pamela Anderson, the truth is much more prosaic. Most of my patients are women who have ended the period of their life that includes childbearing. They may come in as soon as six months or a year after having their last child with their kids in tow or as late as twenty years after their last birth, but their stories always have a common theme. They tell me that the physical changes wrought by pregnancy and nursing, irreparable by diet or exercise, make the "self" they see reflected in the mirror seem unfamiliar. Their drooping, deflated breasts and stretched skin are at odds with the way they feel inside—sexy, vibrant, feminine. They talk of reclaiming the self, not as a way of renouncing their mother-hood, their children, or their choices, but as a way of recapturing an inner identity they've lost and marking that a transition out of one life stage has taken place. This is true even of women who have waited for years to have the surgery; they date wanting the altera-tion to the time they last gave birth. To be sure, some admit to a bit of vanity—that they're looking forward to getting back into a bikini—but what they really want is far more profound. And what do they want? They always put it simply: "I want myself back." That statement takes on special meaning in the context of the early years of mothering, when women often report that the needs of the self are put on protracted hold.

What's amazing to me is how quickly the "self" incorporates the body part transformed; in two or three weeks, my patients will actually feel fully comfortable with their breasts, physically and psy-chologically. Most choose implants that are the same size as their breasts were before pregnancy, and from their point of view, their postsurgical breasts aren't "new." Rather, they are their "old" breasts restored and, in that sense, "theirs." It takes just a few weeks for their preoperative pictures to look strange and foreign.

The need to align the inner vision of the self with the physical body in the mirror appears even more marked in older women who come in seeking facelifts. (Breasts are relatively private, unless you're naked or in a skimpy bathing suit; faces are the most public part of the self.) Even when the motivations for the procedure are different, the patients' narratives tend to fall into the same patterns and are usually connected to a life transition as well. They are less concerned with "pleasing" others than the media coverage of facelifts and aging would suggest. In fact, many of my patients see choosing surgery as a way of laying claim to their bodies in specific ways. The symbolism of the body part they choose to change is usually highly charged with personal meaning.

One woman, not that long ago, came in over her husband's and sons' objections. She clearly saw a facelift as an act of self-assertion and independence, and a redefinition of the role she had played for decades. "I've been taking care of everyone for years," she explained, "husband, sons, household, and family. I am here to take care of myself." She added that while her husband and sons didn't support her choosing surgery, "they've come around to respecting why I want to do this. I will do it with or without them, but with them is better."

For another patient, new changes—a job promotion and a relationship with a younger man—inspired her to want her face to look as energetic and youthful as she felt. The lover, as it happens, didn't care whether she had a facelift or not. Another woman wanted her face to reflect the satisfaction she felt in her life. "Judging from what people say to me, I seem to look tired or angry all the time," she explained, "but I'm not. I want to look the way I feel." There are the women who have been watching their process of aging—and having Botox and other fillers injected—and decide now that it is "time" to have a facelift. There are some who wake up one day—that's how they describe it—and suddenly discover that they are "old." What they all want is to look like "themselves"—the way their inner self feels. Almost always, the decision to have surgery is made in the context of other changes and transitions in the patient's life; it is never random.

My last procedure followed the same pattern. After six years of using Botox on the deep frown line between my eyes, I decided to have a brow and lower-eye lift. Once again, I was attracted by a new endoscopic technique that would yield both natural results and minimal scarring. My decision was spurred on by a transition in my life—turning forty—and a tubal pregnancy that effectively ended the inner discussion I'd had about having a child. Most of my women friends faced this choice as they approached forty, balancing their desire to have a child with both the facts and pressures in their personal and professional lives. I was no exception. I decided to mark this juncture in my life with a lift that would open my own eyes to the world in a different way, both literally and symbolically. This final surgery was a complete success.

As a culture, we tend to distrust these personal narratives for reasons both simple and complicated. But, really, why should we? Why do we insist on believing that these narratives of self are really excuses for vanity or insecurity?

My own anecdotal experience with my patients confirms what one researcher, Kathy Davis, discovered: that the usual reasons women choose to undergo cosmetic surgery—the "why" of it—don't relate in the main to outside forces or unhealthy pressures but very specifically to the storied self and the personal mythology that evolves out of it. First, the stories cosmetic patients told the researcher all followed the same pattern or plotline, beginning with a "before" and an "after" in which the act of having the body surgically altered represented a biographical turning point. Second, each patient saw the surgery as a solution to a problem that had caused her suffering; more important, the patient also saw herself as an active agent in determining the solution. While each narrative also included arguments defending the choice of surgery, Davis surmised that they were simply a reflection of societal ambivalence about cosmetic surgery. Finally, she concluded that each of the narratives was, in fact, a story about identity, and that surgery had helped to "reintegrate" the story of the self.[6]

My own patients' stories follow similar patterns, but how the inner self could be transformed by an external act, wrought by a third party, would only begin to be revealed to me by the experience of a patient who technically didn't have surgery at all.

Years ago, before the word *Botox* passed into the lexicon of everyday life, a young woman in her early thirties visited my office for a consultation. Botox, as everyone now knows, is an inert toxin and most plastic surgeons, myself included, see it as a dunk into the waters of cosmetic surgery, particularly since it is impermanent and thus entails very negligible risk. Except for two very deep frown lines between her eyes—pronounced enough to be visually jarring in a youthful face—she was attractive and articulate. She had just completed her Ph.D. and was about to get married; in short, she was embarking on a fully adult life. She'd come in about the frown lines and asked whether Botox would remove them. I told her one injection alone wouldn't but that after a few, the frown lines would begin to diminish.

I began her treatment that day.

A week later, she unexpectedly returned to my office. She looked totally worn out. Her eyes were red-rimmed and puffy, as if she'd been crying for days which, it turned out, she had been. I was immediately concerned that she'd had an adverse physical reaction to the injections, which is unusual, but even with something as minimally invasive as an injection of Botox, not impossible. When we sat down together, though, she explained that she'd been unable to stop crying in the past few days—that, somehow, when the muscle between her eyes had stopped working, she'd experienced a flood of emotions. Long-forgotten memories of her childhood—of her mother scolding her for not smiling enough, of being told that she looked angry or sad even when she wasn't—suddenly surfaced. "Quit frowning," her mother would say. "You're so pretty when you're smiling." The outpouring of memories—which were so vivid that she actually felt as if she were reliving every incident—in turn released anger and pain.

My patient's experience both amazed and humbled me. How could a single muscle, no larger than a shred of meat caught between the teeth, hold so much information? The directness of the connection—incident upon incident held by a single, tiny part of the body—was astonishing. Her experience hinted at the complexity of the connection between the inner and outer self—the layer upon layer of emotional experience that's held or stored in the physical body—and the ways in which the two interact in the process of healing and wholeness. Her experience was an epiphany for me, and revealed another way in which the body has stories to tell.

If one muscle could hold all that memory, did the body store all of our experiences—almost as if each and every experience had been "written" upon it?

Over time, I have come to see that it is truer than I would have first thought.

While it may seem radical—the idea that the mind and body can interact and change each other—scientific studies have proven that our thoughts can transform our body's chemistry and structure. For example, if we focus our thoughts on the color red, our blood pressure and heart rate will go up; conversely, imagining the color blue will lower both. The placebo effect, well documented in Western medicine, infers that simply thinking that a medication is working enables the physical response without any medicine being given at all. The idea that thoughts can predictably and reliably change measurable physical variables is the basis of the field of biofeedback, which has been proven to give an individual voluntary control over physiological responses. Biofeedback has been proven to be successful in treating chronic pain, some types of insomnia, as well as a number of illnesses.

A growing body of literature supports the effects of visualization and hypnosis before and after surgery, while guided imagery has also been shown to be effective in the treatment of cancer. A technique developed by Francine Shapiro, EMDR (eye movement desensitization and reprocessing), for post-traumatic stress disorder suggests that the information pertaining to trauma is literally stored in the body and can be released by reprocessing that information in other physical ways, specifically by moving the eyes rapidly from side to side while focusing on a segment of traumatic memory. More and more research suggests that the boundaries between the body and the mind are more permeable than absolute; for example, the work of Candace P. Pert has explored the molecular bases of emotions and how they are inseparable from physiology. Long appreciated in non-

Western cultures, the intricate connections between aspects of mind and properties of matter—the body itself—are just beginning to be teased out in the West.[7]

And then there is the body itself and its connection to what we call the "mind." This goes far beyond what we all know by experience—that exercising makes us feel calm, for example, or that tensing our muscles makes us feel uptight. Perhaps no one has written about this relationship as succinctly as Antonio Damasio in his book, *The Feeling of What Happens*. While we tend to think of the mind and body as separate—as Descartes once held—neurobiology teaches a different lesson. Every thought processed by our brain is intrinsically connected to the organism—the body—of which it forms a part. As Damasio explains, the body is the reference point for everything we think, feel, or experience because "whatever happens in your mind happens in time and in space relative to the instant in time your body is in and to the region of space occupied by your body. Things are in or out of you. Those that are out of you are stationary or moving."[8]

Damasio's argument, which begins with this commonsense approach, quickly moves to its logical conclusion, proving simply and irrevocably that there is nothing "pure" about thought or that there is anything that belongs to the mind alone, because the perspective of the body—the physical experience—applies not just to objects in space but to ideas, whether they are abstract or concrete. Individual perspective is always a function of both mind and body."[9]

Seen from this point of view, the things that belong to the self must always involve the body as well.

The experience of my Botox patient opened up new ideas out of old ways of thinking. I already knew that the mind could change the body; what I hadn't fully appreciated was that it seemed equally reasonable to assume that restructuring the body could transform our thoughts and thus change who we are at the deepest level. If what each of us thinks connects directly to the body as a point of reference—whether we classify that thought as "emotional" or "intellectual"—what would happen if the body were significantly changed through surgery? Would our thoughts necessarily change as well?

It was then that I began asking my patients "Why now?" and the patterns of life change and transition began to emerge. And I started to look past the traditional distinctions between elective and non-elective surgery and began to think about surgery as an experience that engaged both the body and the mind. And I wondered what effect the experience of surgery, apart from the results, might have on the individual and her sense of self.

And I began to think about my female patients in a different way. Why were so many of my patients women? The "beauty myth" and other negative social constructs explained why some of them were driven to see me but failed to address the amazingly confident and articulate women who offered very different reasons for wanting to change their bodies. Their narratives of self were rich and compelling, and seemed to hint at explanations very different from the standard answers our society offers about why women seek out elective surgery.

I began to listen to the way the story of a given body part connected to the story of a woman's life and I began to discern a pattern that hinted at an explanation I hadn't thought to consider.

4

Cosmetic Surgery and Rites of Passage

While the tools I use during surgery are distinctly modern, the art I practice is an ancient one. Understanding the larger context of body modification—both in its ancient forms and its modern incarnations—and its relationship to humanity's spiritual growth and longing helps to illuminate the meaning of contemporary cosmetic surgery and offers an answer to the question of why so many women are choosing it. Throughout recorded history, human beings have altered their bodies, seeing flesh and skin both as a creative canvas and a way of marking life passages.

The connection between body modification and rites of passage—those rituals within a society that both affirmed and helped facilitate a change in status or identity for the individual—is universal. Both the predictable transitions of the life cycle—birth, childhood, puberty, marriage, pregnancy, motherhood and fatherhood, death—as well as the unexpected ones such as miscarriage, loss of a loved one, or illness were ritually and symbolically enacted. These rites articulated and gave meaning to the individual life experience and gave it a communal context. Importantly, each life experience was shared and witnessed by others, which gave it universal meaning; nothing important in life was undergone alone.[1]

Each rite was unique, dedicated to a single purpose, and reflected the beliefs and makeup of the culture, but, as a group, rites of passage share distinct characteristics. For example, the life transition from childhood into womanhood with the onset of menarche was universally celebrated by physically removing the girl from her home and immediate family, symbolizing the end of childhood and the beginning of womanhood. She would be cleansed and purified by water or smoke, and would give up the clothes that identified her as a girl and put on garments that symbolized her entry into womanhood. She would be sequestered with female elders at a place specially set aside for that purpose for days or perhaps months, and would be schooled in her adult and female responsibilities. The difficulty of the life transition would then be enacted by a dance that imitated a cosmic journey or a ritual event such as burying the initiate in sand or some other test that symbolized the transitional state. Finally, to signify the change she had undergone, her appearance would be altered in some way, such as by molding a body part, tattooing, or undergoing a rite of scarification, which permanently altered her appearance and, symbolically, her identity.

The way in which body modification worked in these rites of passage was both simple and complex. On the one hand, the changed appearance—the filed-down tooth, the neck elongated by wearing heavy metal rings, the tattooed or scarified breast or face—functioned as an announcement to the world at large that the girl had become a woman and had learned the necessary lessons from her elders. The patterns of tattoos and scars might further identify the girl with a deity or an ancestor or even symbolically connect her new fecundity with that of nature or the earth. The ritual act of filing down teeth—often the canine incisors—could symbolize the release of the initiate's "animal" nature and her transformation as a member of society. But the outside marks also testified to an inner change, which was more profound.

Few of these rituals were without pain or danger, and it's been suggested that the experience of pain—as well as that of fear—was actually central to their performance and meaning. While, on the surface, that may seem counterintuitive, pain and fear also have the effect of intensifying the feeling of being alive. Moreover, both enduring the pain and having the record of it—the scar that is left behind—bear witness to the experience as well as to the change the initiate has undergone. All of these ritual acts assumed that both the girl's outer body and inner being had been transformed.[2]

The experience of pain during the rite of passage, particularly those aimed at girls and boys making the transition into adulthood, also functioned symbolically as preparation for life's positives and negatives, and the universal experiences of both pleasure and pain. In addition, the pain and discomfort experienced during the initiatory ordeal reinforced the internal and external sensation of the presence and power of spirit forces as well as the spiritual life. This aspect of the rites caused religious historian Mircea Eliade to call them the "most significant spiritual phenomena in the history of humanity" because, before undergoing the first rite of passage from childhood to adulthood, each person had not "fully shared in the human condition."[3] Rites of passage were thus an induction into becoming fully human as well as a preparation for the next stage of life and all the stages to follow.

Precisely because these rites were meant to help the individual negotiate a specific life passage successfully, and were to serve as a model for the life transitions to come, pain was often deliberately magnified with acids and other irritants rubbed into raw wounds, for example. The reason behind this may be hard to grasp—why these rites actually magnified pain, rather than reducing it—but, in his seminal book, *The Hero with a Thousand Faces,* Joseph Campbell explained it. Precisely because these rituals were physically violent and extreme, they also forced the mind of the initiate to be "radically cut away from the attitudes, attachments, and life stages of the stage being left behind."[4] In that sense, by suffering through the ordeal, the old self was ritualistically left behind and, by surviving and recovering, the individual was "reborn" into a new stage of life. The extremity of the ordeal—the severity of the fear and pain—engaged the individual on all levels, physical and emotional, conscious and unconscious. The assumption was that without that extreme sever- ance, the individual would be unable to negotiate the transition, and unable to move on to the next stage of life. The physical manifesta- tion of the rite—whether it was a scar, a tattoo, or something else— exemplified the individual's courage and endurance, as well as her ability to withstand the challenges of life. This aspect of the rites may be difficult for us to grasp, since in our twenty-first-century lives, pain is almost universally recognized as a negative experience rather than a facilitative one.

While initiatory rites for boys and males tended to emphasize social roles, those pertaining to girls and women were specifically designed to make the physical and emotional changes in the body visibly manifest, acting as proof that the girl or woman's inner being had been transformed. In one African culture, for example, scars on the area between the breast and the navel would signify a girl's entry into womanhood; a rite celebrating the weaning of her first child would include marks deliberately placed on her back. The body was understood to be symbolic of inner experience, and the marks put on it a map of her life experience. Among the Yoruba people, distinc- tive marks placed on specific parts of the body testified to different experiences, and thus would be recognizable at a glance. The design of the scar—such as that designated as a mark of sorrow—would immediately "tell the story" of the loss of someone dear. In another culture, marks on a woman's calf would testify to her loss of a child through miscarriage. The actual location of scars and marks would reinforce the symbolism of each body part; scars on the abdomen marked fertility, while those on the breasts told the story of child- birth. Each scar, in this sense, represented transitions in life that were permanent and irreversible.[5]

Our bodies still tell stories, but the once-universal language of marking has been lost. In our contemporary society, we have little or no affirmation of the changes we undergo during the life process. Girls get their periods and the event may be hidden in embarrassment or marked by nothing more than handing our daughters a box of pads or tampons and giving them a lecture on sexual responsibility. A driver's license or graduation from high school are but cursory markers of adulthood. After the bridal shower and the wedding, the bride makes the transition from unmarried woman to wife without support or guidance from her community of elders. We give birth in sterile hospitals, often under anesthesia or by C-section, and go home with only self-help books on motherhood to guide us. We experience life transitions such as illness, divorce, and the entry into menopause alone, without the aid of rite or ritual.

What I have found in my work with women is that the needs for ritual and celebration remain with us but have been driven underground, like some half-remembered dream, as numerous scholars and writers have suggested. Mircea Eliade remarks that "initiatory themes and urges remain alive chiefly in the unconscious,"[6] and that would certainly explain why we seem to seek out independent actions and gestures that act as substitutes for the rites that were once an essential part of human self-definition.

I believe that our efforts to modify our bodies through cosmetic surgery and other practices can be better understood in this context. Even though our American culture celebrates the life passages of the individual either superficially or not at all, as a group, we acknowledge that these thresholds or stages of life certainly exist. Bestselling works of nonfiction such as Gail Sheehy's *Passages* and Judith Viorst's *Necessary Losses* have made them part of our popular cultural understanding, but with the possible exceptions of marriage and the birth of a child, the important passages of a woman's life—beginning with menarche—are neither celebrated nor validated in our everyday lives. Still, the need to mark these events physically and psychologically remains with us. Individuals find ways to mark their life transitions, and I believe cosmetic surgery has become one way to do so. As cosmetic surgery becomes more affordable and available, more and more women will turn to it to fill the void left by rite and ritual.

The Cultural Void

At a glance, the connection between cosmetic surgery—something we think of as part of our twenty-first century cornucopia of self-improvement—and ancient rites of passage may seem foreign. For one thing, these rites of passage have largely disappeared from view in most parts of the modern world, suggesting that they are nothing more than historical artifacts of societies less evolved than ours. In addition, the words *rites of passage*, if anything, are likely to summon up images from dusty old issues of *National Geographic:* bare-breasted women with necks deliberately elongated by weights, bodies transformed with circular patterns of scars, villagers with painted faces dancing around a fire in a faraway place. These images seem as far removed from our fast-moving contemporary American life as those of distant planets—interesting, perhaps, but hardly relevant.

Consciously or not, we wrap ourselves in the mantle of progress, secure in the knowledge that our culture is more enlightened, more scientific, more evolved than any of those "primitive" societies that wielded knife or sharpened stone to mark the body in honor of life's passages.

What this vision of modern enlightenment and our pride in historical forward motion assume is that we as humans are different in some important sense from those who came before us. We feel not only separate but superior to those who, in our eyes at least, believed in the "magic" of transformation.

But—and it is a very big and important "but"—just as the cycle of human life has stayed the same, encompassing a journey from birth to death, so, too, have the humans living it. We may have more varied and nutritious diets, stay healthier, and live longer more comfortably and easily than our ancestors, but there is something about our humanity that has stayed immutable. We read literature written hundreds and thousands of years ago for this reason, and pore over sculptures and paintings from ancient civilizations not just to learn about our forebears but to learn about ourselves. And precisely because the human condition—the being born, the growing, the living, the dying, and the connecting and the separating—has stayed constant, the need for ritual process bubbles up out of a primal impulse, revealing itself in patterns that coexist in our modern lives alongside our denial of them.

Whether we are aware of them or not, these patterns also permeate our popular culture; they are present in the movies and television shows we watch, the novels and magazine articles we read. Carl Jung, who has greatly influenced my thinking about cosmetic surgery, provided the philosophical groundwork for explaining how mythology the world over expresses a universal pattern closely connected to initiatory rites.[7] In these myths, a person or hero suffers a crisis and is separated from all he or she knows; suffers physical pain or is thrust into a place of suffering; and, in the end, reemerges whole as a new person transformed or reborn. The myths' ubiquity suggests, indeed, that the human beings may be "hardwired" to process experience in this three-part cycle, for as Robert Moore writes, "The structure is paradigmatic to human experience. We all go through this night sea journey many times in our lives, with some journeys smaller and less dangerous than others, but it is still the same cycle over and over again."[8] Mirea Eliade also comments that the pattern of initiation is so embedded in the human psyche that our stories and experiences echo it over and over.[9] These narrative patterns animate contemporary novels with male and female heroes and heroines, self-help narratives, memoirs, as well as the stories we tell our friends, because the human condition remains the same. With little variation the framework of these narratives—the sudden awakening that comes from a turn in life—shows up in magazine articles and on television as well.

In the last century, Jung's writings and, more popularly, those of Joseph Campbell suggested that the similarity and ubiquity of myths and mythic patterns across the globe revealed a commonality of inherited ways of thinking or archetypal ideas that have existed in every human mind. In this century, science, with its newly enhanced ability to study the different parts of the brain, has suggested that human mythmaking and the need for ritual may have a neurological basis—that, indeed, we may be hardwired for these experiences in a much more literal way than Jung or Campbell ever suspected. As the authors of *Why God Won't Go Away* write, "Myths are created by the basic, universal aspects of the brain, in particular the fundamental process through which the brain makes sense of the world. Although culture and psychology may influence them significantly, it's the neurological grounding of mythic stories that gives them their staying power."[10]

But even though the cycle of life experience retains its basic pattern and our need for ritual and myth remains constant, our contemporary culture retains only the bare remnants of what was once a supportive framework for giving it meaning.

Women's Bodies, Women's Rites

I have come to see that there are reasons beyond the cultural pressures that might explain why women, more than men, choose to alter their bodies through surgery. We all know and recognize that women and men inhabit their bodies differently, in part because female biology doesn't easily permit us to see our bodies as mere "envelopes" encasing the self. While hormone secretions influence perceptions and emotions in both men and women, the constant cycle of those changes in the female body makes our awareness of them different in kind. We understand and experience the connection between mind and body in myriad ways from the very first time we get our periods and pass out of the androgyny of childhood into a female body and self. The changes in our female bodies from puberty onward are grounded in time, and our perception of the self, throughout our adulthood, is shaped by the process.

Women's bodies bear witness to the passages of female experiences and the changing self in ways that male bodies, with a simpler reproductive system, do not. As females, we confront and are confronted by our bodies in very specific ways—ways that belie the distinction between the inner self and the outer shell. There is a very specific sense in which our female identity—as contrasted with that of a man—is indeed embodied.

Emerging from childhood, we grow breasts and hips and, most important, begin to bleed. We may suffer from premenstrual syndrome, bloating, and cramping on a monthly basis; we may feel tired or down or cranky. The body—the fleshly vehicle through which we feel—is also an active participant in how we feel, day to day, week to week, month to month—an experience that isn't shared by men. The neurochemical pathways in our brains are changed by the fluctuations in estrogen and progesterone levels, which, in turn, affect both our emotions and our perceptions of ourselves and the world around us.

On reflection, no woman would have proposed mind-body dualism because it wouldn't have made any sense.

The relationship between the female self and the body is an ongoing one, and certain of the life passages—such as motherhood—are experienced physically by the female of our species alone. Once again, physical and emotional changes go hand in hand. Childbearing changes the shape of our bodies, the size of our hands and feet, the texture of our hair and skin, just as the flood of hormones shapes our thoughts and feelings by changing the pathways in the brain. Nursing is another passage experienced both physically and emotionally.

Similarly, perimenopause and then menopause, whether we have borne children or not, bring changes that force us to confront the end of our childbearing years and the fact of our aging in ways that are both physical and emotional. We cease menstruating; our skin and ligaments become less elastic, our bones more fragile. We may suffer mood swings, hot flashes, as well as sleeplessness; we may become more forgetful, and the decline in our estrogen levels may make us more vulnerable to depression. While men continue to be able to father children, our female bodies don't allow us to deny our aging; we feel the changes as we see them.

For all of the culture's emphasis on the surface of the female body—the trim thigh, the firm breast, the sculpted derriere—we each know that the body as we experience it from the inside actively forms and shapes the self. The female body and the female self are partners in an intricate dance with identifiable stages or passages.

Yet in our modern culture it is a dance without music, accompaniment, or a setting, performed alone, without support. In premodern societies, the stages of a woman's life were articulated by the acknowledgment of inner changes with outer-body modification. These rites put the individual experience into a meaningful and symbolic cultural context, affirming the identities of all those involved.

While it may seem radical, most of the women who come into my office—whether they are fully conscious of the underlying motivation or not—seek both physical transformation as well as physical affirmation of an internal change that has either taken place or is about to. Women about to get married or women who have been through a divorce. Women who have recently cared for an ill or dying loved one. Women who themselves have survived a life-threatening illness. Women whose children have recently left the nest. Women who have been fired from their jobs or received a promotion. Women who have just entered menopause. Women who have just entered a new decade of life.

Within these broad patterns are individual responses to the

transition at hand. The young woman in her twenties, suddenly and cruelly widowed, who came in for breast augmentation. Shortly after her surgery, she found a new partner and is now expecting a child. The woman in her forties whose hooded and drooping eyelids—a familial legacy—no longer expressed her lightness of being. Her life had been marked by pivotal changes—illness and surgery, the end of a long-term relationship, the completion of a doctorate—and she wanted her eyes to reflect the changes within her. The woman in her sixties who came in to discuss breast reduction, something she'd been thinking about since she'd nursed her children thirty years ago. When I asked her, "Why now?"—the question I ask all of my patients—she painted a picture of a life so stable, so lacking in a significant landmark change, that I thought I must have missed something. I wasn't surprised, however, when, on her next visit, she moved the date of her surgery so that she could fly to another city to welcome her first grandchild into the world.

The pattern of patients' responses remains the same from week to week, year to year, whether it was the woman who came to see me on the tenth anniversary of her mother's death, the patient who came in for a facelift within a month of resolving a long and difficult family lawsuit, or the woman who called impatient for an appointment after years of waiting to have her nose, damaged in a fall, repaired right before her fortieth birthday.

Over and over, my patients' own stories attest to the urgent need to make life passages physically manifest, laying claim to the experience on the body in the same way an adolescent girl may pierce her umbilicus not just as a fashion statement but as a symbolic way of redefining her relationship to her mother. Just recently I got a call from a woman any one of us would easily and readily identify as strong, independent, and not easily swayed by societal pressures. Long married, she bore her three children late. She is forty-five and her call was occasioned both by the recent weaning of what she knows to be her last child and the entry of her eldest daughter into adolescence. "I'm in a significant mourning period," she told me, "now that I know that I am too old to have more children. My husband loves me the way I am, but I've decided to have a breast lift and a facelift as a way to mark my moving on." These, by the way, are the words of a health-conscious Californian who neither wears makeup nor dyes her hair.

Each story revealed the complexity of the need for ritual marking. That need was connected to acts of commemoration, mourning, and, sometimes, closure. The woman whose early life was marked by her mother's suicide and who decided to have a tummy tuck when she reached her mother's age at the time of her death. The woman who had been left devastated and desperate after the death of her only child and came to me feeling guilty about wanting something that seemed so superficial—a facelift— in the wake of tragedy. Importantly, her husband had encouraged her, and had seen that choosing to change herself physically was an act of reclamation in the aftermath of terrific loss. For her, choosing surgery was both a way to remember her grief and, paradoxically, to let go of it. Sometimes the symbolism of the surgery is open and transparent. One woman came in asking for a breast lift and a tummy tuck. Her child had been stillborn and she was unable to speak about her loss without weeping. I advised her to wait a year, which she did. She returned on the anniversary of her child's birth and death, and symbolically restored her body to wholeness. She conceived a child successfully shortly thereafter and gave birth to a healthy baby.

Sometimes the decision to undergo surgery is a celebration of a life transition or crisis successfully forded. There was the patient, a single mother, who had wanted breast augmentation for years but had put it off while she struggled with her daughter's abuse of drugs. She decided to have the surgery after her child successfully completed drug rehabilitation and became healthy and clean. A woman facing sixty scheduled an eye and a facelift just before her birthday. As a single career woman who had never married or had children, her gift to herself was also a symbolic act. "I am doing this to celebrate myself," she said, "and I can hear my mother, who always took care of herself and who celebrated me, cheering in heaven."

Choosing surgery can also be a symbolic act of restoration. One patient had open heart surgery as a child and had one undeveloped breast as a result. She came to me for an augmentation when she decided she needed to leave her childhood behind and move into her adult future. A year after the surgery, she was married and expecting a child. Breast reduction lifts the physical weight off a woman's shoulders, but it may also reflect a symbolic weight as well. One of my patients developed large breasts after childbirth and nursing but her decision to have the surgery was finally triggered by her youngest child's moving out, when she could symbolically unload the "weight" of motherhood.

Even more telling, roughly half of my breast reconstruction patients, survivors of cancer, come back to have elective surgery, either at the completion of their treatment or to mark their recovery on a significant anniversary—five or ten years—after their initial diagnosis. The symbolism of choosing elective surgery is perhaps most evident for these women, whose initial surgery entailed no choice and was a rite of passage out of health into illness and then into healing. The "willing wound"—the surgery entered into by choice—is different in kind, is highly symbolic, and entails a real sense of agency.

Once I understood, almost ten years ago, that choosing cosmetic surgery was closely linked to the need for ritual, I began to see that surgery—whether elective or not—is, in and of itself, a rite of passage that leaves the patient changed in profound ways that go beyond the changes on the surface of the body. I also realized that contemporary surgery—in both its structure and its effects—mirrors and mimics the structure and effect of initiatory and other rites closely enough to provide some of the benefits of the body and self changed through ritual experience.

In this context, the submission to the surgical process, the surgical wound, the experience of recovery, the healing and the scar it leaves behind become part of the process of the personal acknowledgment of inner transformation.

Rites of Passage and Inner Growth

The connection between personal growth and the physical aspect of initiation was profound and important. As Michael Meade writes, the physical pain experienced by the initiate—through wounding, scarring, or piercing—not only "severs" her from her past self but forcibly begins the process of evolving a new self. As such, the blood that is let or exposed during a rite "represents the immediate, mutual presence of life and death" in literal and symbolic terms. Through wounding, the old self is killed and the new self, hidden within, is permitted to emerge.[11]

The formal rites that once celebrated life transitions no longer exist, but the requirement that we let go of our former selves to move on to the next stage of life still remains, and the transitions we experience are no easier than they were for our ancestors. In her book *Necessary Losses,* which never mentions initiatory rites but describes patterns that are identical, Judith Viorst writes, "These losses are part of life—universal, unavoidable, inexorable. And these losses are necessary because we grow by losing and leaving and letting go." Gain, Viorst tells us, is impossible without loss; in order to grow, we must also give up. Beginning in childhood, we must constantly redefine ourselves as our bodies change, as the events in our personal lives shape us, and as the way in which others perceive us shifts. Inevitably, the life journey requires that we give up parts of our old identities and move on to new definitions of self. This process is never easy and is, inevitably, filled with pain as we move from the familiar and safe to the unknown and the new, and we give up old ties to forge new relationships.[12]

Popular psychology, too, acknowledges that spiritual and psychological growth cannot be accomplished without risk, loss, and pain. In his best-selling book *The Road Less Traveled*, M. Scott Peck made much the same point, though he focused on what happens to people when they try to avoid the knowledge that life and death are linked and that, as he put it, "the further one travels on the journey of life, the more births one will experience—and therefore the more deaths—the more joy and the more pain."[13]

But even though the process of human growth remains the same, in our contemporary society we don't have either a social context in which we can experience those losses as necessary or a physical way of processing them. If we mourn these losses, we largely mourn alone. We move from one stage of life to another in isolation, acting as though the mind-body split were real. In contrast, the ancient rites of passage and initiations required that the passage be experienced both psychically and physically within a communal setting. Since the mind and body were understood to be one, changing the mind without changing the body—pulling the individual's mind and the individual's body forcibly into the next stage of experience—was unthinkable.

These rites of passage included steps and stages that made the separation of the individual from where he or she was in life physically and emotionally manifest. First, the individual was literally separated from communal life—from his or her dwelling, as well as from the center of communal space. In addition, the individual was ritually purified, by stripping away both the clothing and support that signified the loss of his or her place or status in life, as well as his or her earlier identity. The initiate was stripped down to his or her essential nature. Purification—usually by fasting—was yet another part of the process of severing ties to what had come before. Next, the individual was required to enter a sacred space—a place set physically apart from the ordinary locales of life—voluntarily. In terms of ritual symbolism, this indicated the individual's willingness to surrender to the process of change and transformation. Because all of these symbolic changes were also experienced physically, they imitated the very process that transformation entails. Victor Turner has called this liminal space—the space that is at the "threshold"— indicating that the initiate is without moorings of identity and is poised to be remade.[14]

It is at that point in the ritual process that the separation or severance from the previous life stage is made physically manifest, by cutting or marking the body. Surrendering to the pain of the marking was both literal and symbolic, as the individual submitted him- or herself to the process of transformation. It is at that moment of ultimate separation and intense physical feeling (pain) that the next stage of life begins. The initiate would return to society when his or her wounds were healed, and the scars testified to the change within.

Surgery imitates these steps almost precisely.

The patient leaves the outside world behind, is cleansed and purified by antibacterial showers and scrubs, and cut loose from all that is familiar, thus beginning the unmooring and dismantling of the self. She removes the garment of outer life which symbolizes her identity. When she enters the inner sanctum of the operating room, she is separated from those who care about her. She voluntarily submits to lying down on the operating table—a modern-day altar—and then undergoes a death/rebirth sequence that, in its contemporary form, is anesthesia. Her body is marked, wounded, and transformed. She wakes to acknowledge her wounds and begins the journey toward wholeness.

For those who haven't undergone surgery, understanding it as a process and an experience is essential to choosing it.

There are two operating rooms, one experienced by the surgeon and the other by the patient whether or not the surgery is elective or the result of illness. Like the sacred space in which a rite of passage was performed, the operating room is deliberately, ritualistically set apart from the larger world of everyday society. Both surgeon and patient are required to act in ways that openly acknowledge the room's separation from the world outside. It is a universe unto itself, a hierarchy with carefully defined roles and a choreography of steps and actions, all of which simultaneously impose order on the surgical process and acknowledge its dangers and risks.

From the surgeon's point of view—and that of the staff in the operating room—those risks, though not center stage, are ever-present. Surgery offers reminders, in the simplest and most humbling ways, that nothing in this life is stable or totally predictable, and the rituals of the operating room are meant to keep the dangers inherent in the process at bay. For example, sponges, sutures, and the like—objects that can be left in the patient's body by accident—are counted and recounted ritually and meaningfully during the course of an operation. I am mentally prepared for the unexpected despite the routines of surgery because each case is different and anomalies happen. My awareness is heightened, as is that of my patient. In this sense, too, the operating room is like the sacred space of ritual, for as Robert L. Moore notes, the ritual elders knew that transformative space was fragile and they couldn't control it; they approached it with deep humility, not arrogance.[15]

As the surgeon, I take off the clothes that connect me to my roles in the outer world—friend, lover, sister, daughter, aunt—and put on the androgynous blue or green scrubs that declare my identity and status as the doctor. I put on rubber clogs, which can easily be wiped clean of blood. My hair is covered, my face masked, and my eyes protected from blood transmission and corrected for the close-up work of surgery. Whoever I am in the outside world has been deliberately hidden from view, and my separation from the larger world is almost complete.

In rites of passage, the elder or elders who performed the ritual were similarly anointed and cleansed, taking on the role of teacher, guide, and facilitator.

Like the initiate in a rite of passage, the patient has undergone her own journey of separation, leaving her everyday life behind. She has planned for this event, putting the ordinary rhythms of life on hold. She has arranged for her own care after surgery, as well as the needs of her family and employer, thus acknowledging the disruption that surgery represents. She has undergone a rite of purification, having eaten nothing since the night before and having washed her hair and body with antibacterial soap that morning. She has arrived at the hospital early, usually accompanied by a friend or relative, to fill out reams of paperwork, which help to bring the surgery into the now of the present. She has had to let go of all the things that identify her in the world outside—her keys, wallet, purse, cell phone, and jewelry are all relinquished. If she is having facial surgery, she has taken off her makeup. She takes off her clothing and puts on a hospital gown that barely covers her. And then, still in the company of friends or family, she waits.

It is usually a transition period of high stress and anxiety as she awaits a journey into the unknown, just as it was for the initiate, who anticipated the danger and rigor that lay ahead.

She takes leave of her loved ones and walks or is wheeled into the operating theater, the inner sanctum of the hospital. She waits to meet the anesthesiologist and then, when I arrive, we talk about the surgery and its goals. This serves as reconfirmation of her conscious choice to have her body altered surgically. If her surgery involves the body, I will ask the men in the room to leave. She disrobes and stands naked before me as I mark her skin with a black pen in preparation. She then lies down on the operating table, which is hard and narrow and sometimes cold, like the stone altars used in many rites.

Breast surgery requires that the patient's arms be arranged at ninety-degree angles to the body and positioned on boards with towels so that, during the course of the operation, she can be placed in a sitting position—this way I can make her breasts look as natural as possible when she is upright. The irony of this Christ-like position of sacrifice is rarely lost on the patient, and helps to ease the tension she feels at this moment.

The patient is at the center of the room, lying still in a sea of motion. While the surrender is not yet complete, she must give herself over to the process and the hands of the professionals who surround her. Anesthesia is the part of the process almost all of my patients fear most. For most, it represents the unknown, and losing consciousness is the ultimate loss of control and surrender. Symbolically, it is a stand-in for the greater fear that lurks beneath every surgery, the fear of death, and directly parallels the fear and uncertainty faced by the initiate in a rite of passage. This part of the surgery also echoes that moment in a rite of passage when the initiate willingly surrenders to the ritual process.

The anesthesiologist starts the monitors and begins to administer medication as I stroke the patient's arm or hold her hand. I ask her to think about a relaxing place—a beach or mountaintop—or somewhere she feels safe and happy. Many patients will visualize the people they love. It is important to her healing that the image in her mind be safe and sustaining. This juncture in surgery has its parallel in the moment when the initiate gives him- or herself over to the process.

I leave the operating room and go to the sink. The handwashing is ritualistic and precise as I scrub at the nails and fingers of my hands, one at a time, for three minutes, allowing the water to drip down my arms and onto my elbows; it is an ablution in the truest sense, similar in kind and intention to ritual uses of water in ceremony and rite. I am to be rendered immaculate. I might be alone at the sink or surrounded by other surgeons, but the act of hand-washing reinforces the break between all the everyday subjects of chatter and the start of the surgery. Ceremonial ablution connects to both body and spirit, and while the cleansing of hands before surgery is intended to prevent incidental bacterial infection, its ritual nature, its repetitions, its deliberateness, and its duration have the effect of cleansing in another sense as well. My mind empties of the minutiae of daily life, readying me for the concentration surgery demands. Just as my hands are clean, so is my intention pure, for the injunction of the physician is always "Do no harm."

I have touched the last things I will touch before touching the patient's body, and walk into the operating room with my hands elevated and dripping. The scrub nurse hands me a towel to dry my hands and then holds up a blue paper gown. I put my hands through the armholes, making sure I do not touch anything. My hands are gloved by the nurse. Whoever I am in the outside world has been transformed and distilled. Should anyone touch me, by accident or on purpose, I will consider myself no longer immaculate, and will have to start over.

The light in the operating room is otherworldly, diffuse but with bright lights over the operating table. The twenty-first century has filled the room with sound, separate from that of human voices or footfalls; the beeping and humming of monitors and machines underline the separation of this room from the regular world in which we live. Their sound reminds me and everyone in the room that we are to be watchful and careful. The instruments are lined up neatly on trays, with the handles facing the surgical field; they are sharp, gleaming, sterile. The patient is asleep on the table, and I begin to drape her with towels and, later, blue cloths that separate the parts of the body that will be left untouched during surgery from those to be transformed. The areas to be cut are painted in Betadine—cleansing them, marking them, separating them from the other parts of the body. This, too, is done carefully, ritualistically.

As I lift up the scalpel toward the body part, which has become abstract—a surgical site rather than the flesh of a living person—I try to become present in the moment, taking a deep breath. I get a surge of adrenaline even though I have done this thousands of times before. The first incision with the scalpel is spoken out loud and noted by the anesthesiologist on his or her record. The operation has begun.

The first drops of blood flow freely. The bovie (cautery) settings are adjusted and the smell of burning flesh suffuses the room. The nurses scramble to suck the toxic smoke from the air. I've grown used to the smell and dislike the distraction their movement creates as I focus entirely on the surgical site.

My actions, after years of experience, are quick and predictable as I get into the flow of the surgery. The music I play when I operate helps me get into it, and I experience a sense of heightened awareness. The act of molding the flesh is a creative one, drawing on all my senses but, most particularly, that of touch. Flesh is removed, weighed, then discarded, or sent to pathology.

The anatomy under my hands has become deeply familiar over the years, making me more sensitive to the small differences—the blood vessel hardened by aging, the distended veins of a woman who has lost a lot of weight. I can both see these differences and feel them, since I wear the thinnest, most sensitive gloves I can.

There is a union that takes place during the operation, a connection between the body of my patient and my own. I work with love and respect, trusting my intuition, letting my hands and eyes inform me of the process. There is, at these moments, an intimate bond between us.

I am aware that she will wake in pain and I put local anesthetic in the wound to lessen it, but I also know that the pain itself cannot be avoided. Pain is part of the healing process; the wounded body will rally its strength to begin the journey back to wholeness. With the last suture in place, the operation ends.

My work is done. The patient's is just beginning; for her, the journey into wholeness can also be a doorway or portal to inner transformation.

As the poet Rumi wrote: "Don't turn your head / Keep looking at the bandaged place / That is where the light enters you."[16]

Filling the Void: The Need for Ritual Marking

I believe the rise in cosmetic surgeries is also connected to the parallel trends of tattooing and piercings—related forms of body modification—among the young, most particularly adolescents making the transition into adulthood and young adults experiencing their first major life passage. While this phenomenon is often explained in terms of contemporary fashion or rebellion, it, too, has its underpinnings in a yearning for ritual marking as well as a need to have the body reflect the inner self or identity during the first of the life transitions. Not surprisingly, women at another stage—the passage of midlife—have also turned to tattooing as a way of marking the transition. It's worth saying that while tattooing is often associated with outsider status, these women are those we would all label as otherwise conventional.[17]

Tattooing and piercing "mark" both the event of passage as well as the body itself, connecting the interior and exterior, the self and the body, in a literal and visual way. For example, in the wake of September 11, the *New York Times* reported on the many individuals who—in reponse to the events of that day—chose to mark their bodies with commemorative tattoos. Historian Jane Caplan rightly connected these tattoos as being part of a continuum from "the yellow ribbons to the spontaneous shrines of flowers that spring up when young people are killed. When these things fill in for the lack of other rituals, they become the rituals by which society commemorates events that are traumatic and fills a space which is empty."[18]

In that sense, cosmetic surgery can also be seen as filling in "an empty space" in the fabric of society. It is part of a continuum of practices of body modification that intend to make the experiences of the "inner self" visible on the "outside" body. Susan Benson has written that all body modifications are linked by a common process

that includes "the piercing of the skin, the flow of blood, the inflic-
tion of pain" and then "the healing of the wound and the visible
trace of this process of penetration and closure." Benson stresses that
body modification is primarily a symbolic act, and that this way of
transforming the flesh can also be understood as a "rich and complex
meditation on issues of agency, autonomy, and control." Personal
narratives make it equally clear that pain as well as the permanence
of the mark are part of the individuation that tattooing and piercing
offer; as one person put it, "If there had been no pain, then the tattoo
on my shoulder might as well have been house paint."[19]

Cosmetic surgery—with its piercing, blood, pain, healing, and
scarring—can also be seen as a symbolic act, which can, indeed,
transform more than the outer body and articulate changes within
the self. Acquiring a "willing wound"—one that has been chosen for
the self—is also part of the transformative process, just as undergoing a rite of passage willingly once was.

Substitute Behaviors and the Loss of Ritual

The hole left in the fabric of our communal life by the loss of ritual
echoes across the cultural landscape. It's been suggested that addictions, violence, and even gang activity are all inadequate substitutes
for human needs and impulses once fully articulated and channeled
by rites of passage and initiation. Over two decades ago, psycho-
analyst Marion Woodman, writing about America's struggles with
addictions—most particularly food and alcohol—observed that in
the absence of what she called a "collective container for their natural spiritual growth," people's need for "transcendent experience, for
ritual, for connection to some greater energy than their own" was
"distorted" into addictive behavior.[20] Others have suggested that
many categories of psychopathology—particularly during the years

of adolescence—may be understood as failed or incomplete initiations. Gangs and their activity—which usually include some form of violent initiation—can also be seen through this lens.[21]

More specifically, the absence of female rituals in our contemporary culture may also explain why women in greater numbers and with greater frequency than men engage in varied practices of body modification, as they satisfy the needs felt at life transitions by other means. Individual narratives about body modification in its myriad forms confirm that women understand their bodies to be intimately connected to the inner self and vehicles for expressing changes in that inner self. The broad spectrum of body modification includes tattooing, piercing, and cosmetic surgery as well as destructive and aberrant behaviors such as cutting and self-mutilation and eating disorders. Just as the preponderance of cosmetic surgery patients are women, the sufferers of practices that are unhealthy substitutes for ritual—self-injury and disordered eating—are also preponderantly female.

In her book, *The Hungry Self: Women, Eating, and Identity*, Kim Chernin made the radical suggestion that the disappearance of the rite of passage at puberty—the purpose of which was "to move the individual from an earlier phase in the life cycle, to separate her from childhood, and make possible the movement into the next stages of development" as well as to "awaken the individual to a sense of social and collective responsibility"—was connected to the rise in disordered eating among adolescent girls, and the obsession so many women have with food. In fact, Chernin stated categorically that an "eating disorder coincides with an underlying developmental crisis, regardless of a woman's age."[22]

Rites of passage were, of course, meant to address and aid the individual in negotiating these developmental crises. Chernin pointed out that girls and women suffering from disorders display both ritualistic behavior pertaining to food and eating, as well as "significant ceremonial intention." She saw these behaviors as the result of women responding to a "cultural lack," thus evolving "some fragmentary and incomplete form of this rite of passage." This effort is doomed, in Chernin's opinion, because "much of the obsessive quality of an eating disorder arises precisely from the fact that food is being asked to serve a transformative function it cannot carry by itself."[23]

Even as Chernin acknowledged the meaningful differences between contemporary food obsessions and "the deliberately, fully involved ceremonies of earlier cultures," she speculated that because rites of passage were necessary for many different stages of life—not just adolescence, when eating disorders tend to develop in our culture—the moment at which eating disorders began to trouble women in other age groups would be a sign that "we are in urgent need of a ceremonial form to guide us beyond what well may be the collective childhood of female identity into a new maturity of female social development."[24]

The Hungry Self was published in 1985, and Chernin's observations have recently proved to be prescient. In the last few years, it has become clear both through research and anecdotal reporting that eating disorders are indeed rising among women in midlife—a new and surprising phenomenon. In March of 2003, Ginia Bellafante reported in the *New York Times*, in an article titled "When Midlife Seems Just an Empty Plate," on the rising number of middle-aged women who had either experienced a relapse of adolescent eating disorders or were experiencing eating disorders for the first time. As Bellafante wrote, "The anxieties of midlife—divorce, marital strains, parental deaths, empty-nest syndrome, and menopause—are powerful catalysts for older women's eating disorders."[25]

Eating disorder clinics all over the country have reported a similar rise in disorders among middle-age women, prompting the Renfrew Center Foundation to devote the Summer 2004 issue of its journal *Perspectives* to what it called "a relatively new and so far rarely explored topic in our field—eating disorders and midlife."

The journal noted that the majority of new patients were thirty-five and older—the age bracket that coincides, not surprisingly, with the highest concentration of women who seek out cosmetic surgery. As two experts, Sandra Kronberg and Vicki Paley, noted, with the onset of an eating disorder, fears and anxieties about life are "translated" into fears and worries about body and weight. And while many of the fears induced by life cannot be controlled, those about body and weight can be. In that sense, "the eating disorder becomes the voice of that which is too painful, frightening, or deep to be put into words. The eating disordered voice and language becomes a powerful coping mechanism and creative adaptation for survival."[26] In the new millennium, in the absence of ritual, women turn instead to substitutes that cannot effect true transformation but which act as stopgap measures in times of transitional crisis.

In a similar vein, Dr. Kathryn J. Zerbe, one of the nation's leading experts on disordered eating and one of the first to report the phenomenon of mid- and late-life eating disorders, used Judith Viorst's idea of "necessary losses" to explain it. She wrote that midlife eating disorders are a defense against the inevitable losses entailed in this life transition, including but not limited to the loss of a youthful body and appearance, changes in the primary relationships with one's own parents, spouse, and children, and particular goals and career aspirations.[27] Without a mechanism to grieve or mourn these losses publicly and meaningfully, some women in midlife substitute the body modification and sense of control offered by disordered eating.

This new research on eating disorders confirmed what I had already seen in my own practice: that the need to have the body reflect and make manifest the life passage remained a primal impulse, which would bubble up in our society in unexpected ways.

Similarly, the rise in the number of self-injurers or cutters may also represent individual answers to a crisis of transition. In their book, *Bodily Harm*, Karen Conterio and Wendy Lader point out that managing emotions and making internal emotional pain manifest in external pain are central to self-mutilation. They note that "our patients often say that their scars tell their life's history. Each scar represents a particularly important event that the patient does not want to forget."[28] The role that the scar plays in the cutter's life is similar to that of the more benign commemorative tattoo; as Susan Benson puts it, "Again, what is external is transformed into something internal to the subject; and memory, a critical property of contemporary self-identity, is externalized and fixed upon the skin."[29] The parallels between this aberrant modern phenomenon and ancient rites of scarification are clear.

Individuals suffering from body dysmorphic disorder (BDD), another disease that has its onset during the first of the major life transitions of adolescence and early adulthood, also turn to body modification as a way of soothing their distress, though to little effect. Although the etiology of BDD remains unknown, it has been suggested that it may be "a pathological response to the various physical and physiological changes of adolescence." Research on BDD is, as Katherine Phillips, M.D., writes, "still in its infancy"; it was only formally classified as a mental disorder, largely unreported but relatively common, less than a decade ago. Typically, BDD is accompanied by obsessive ritualistic behavior pertaining to the perceived defect, such as the patient constantly comparing herself to others, repeatedly checking the perceived flaw in mirrors, grooming excessively, seeking reassurance about the perceived defect, and camouflaging the flaw with hair or clothing. These rituals are extremely time-consuming and effectively take over the individual's life. While this ritualized behavior is usually performed privately, some sufferers will make the behaviors communal as they encourage family and friends to participate—holding up mirrors or lights to the defect, measuring body parts and the like. Almost one-third of women and men with BDD pick their faces compulsively to rid themselves of the defect, resulting in scars and lesions. Other compulsive rituals include excessive exercise, repeating gestures that have "magical" or "ritual" significance, such as washing hands or touching doorknobs, and ritualistic praying.[30]

Individuals with BDD often become "polysurgery addicts," seeking out the ultimate surgery either to "fix" the perceived defect or to alter another body part in order to deflect attention from the perceived defect. While it's been estimated that some 6 to 15 percent of individuals seeking out elective cosmetic surgery suffer from BDD, one thing is clear: They will be neither satisfied by the results nor transformed by the experience, no matter how many surgeries they have.[31] While no researcher has yet suggested a connection between BDD and the modern loss of rites of passage, the ritualized aspects of the disorder are noteworthy, as is the timing of its onset, during adolescence and early adulthood. In addition, BDD effectively stops the transition to a new stage of life, just as anorexia reverts the physical development of the female body and returns it to childhood. Because of their preoccupying behavior, individuals with BDD remain stuck in time: Dr. Phillips notes that some 41 percent of her adult patients still live with their parents, are unemployed, haven't graduated from school, and do not interact socially with others. Seventy-five percent of them never marry or form intimate relationships.[32]

It may well be that all these disorders are substitute behaviors formed in answer to the crisis of life transition in our culture. Christina Grof has suggested that we create our "own pseudorites of passage without knowing it" when we confront an environment that neither appreciates the significance of our ongoing life cycles nor "provides a sanctioned framework for their expression." She notes that these substitutes are either superficial or self-destructive and "are usually projected outward so that there is little or no awareness of their possible effect."[33] Considering people who physically harm themselves during transition states, Robert L. Moore writes that "some theorists just view this as a failure of the human machine. But if you believe that people evolved so that the ritual process is *necessary* to be human, and that we are wired to seek out initiatory process, then such mutilating behaviors may indicate fragmented attempts to start a process leading to a transformation or metamorphosis of the ego to a higher, more mature state. . . . The psyche is trying to do what it needs to do, but there is no one there to dance with, no ritual elder to instruct them in an appropriate healing response to the promptings of the psyche."[34]

One thing not yet addressed by science is that all of these pathological substitutes literally and symbolically stop life transitions from taking place. The anorexic adolescent ceases menstruating and her curves melt away, and she returns to girlhood at least symbolically; the anorexic in middle age turns away from the questions raised by the life passage at hand and retreats into focusing on controlling her body. The woman or man with BDD remains suspended in time, retracing her or his steps again and again to a different physician's office.

While these behaviors may be unconscious replacements for rites of passage our culture no longer provides, they actually perform the opposite function.

Surgery as a Rite of Passage

Ironically, the way our culture frames the dialogue about cosmetic surgery has prevented us from seeing its potential as a tool for transformation as well as its real effect on the individual. Both sides—for and against—have minimized the surgical process, which is at the heart of the matter. Proponents of cosmetic surgery trivialize the risk, the pain, the recovery, and the scarring—even though the patient will experience them all with great intensity. Similarly, by insisting on the "superficiality" of the change offered by cosmetic surgery, opponents equally ignore the very real effects of the experience of surgery itself.

But surgery—*any* surgery, elective or not—encompasses all of the stages and steps that were once a part of ancient rites of passage and, like them, represents a crisis or turning point for the individual. These remarkable similarities give cosmetic surgery, when undergone by an adult acting with agency and awareness, the potential to transform the individual inside and out.

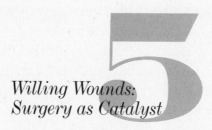

Willing Wounds:
Surgery as Catalyst

The day after surgery, I will see my patient when she is suffering the worst of the pain she will experience; hurting and often nauseated, she will be medicated, on Demerol or morphine, with drainage tubes collecting blood from the surgical site. This is, for most patients, a difficult passage where the carefully constructed and controlled outer self seems besieged, fragmented by the intrusive hospital routines, the isolation of the wounded self, the intensity of feeling. Defenses come down under fire, and it's not unusual for a patient to express doubt about having chosen surgery. "Why did I do this to myself?" is a question that sometimes rises out of the pain and the bandages. Alternatively, she may feel intensely needy or alone.

The comforting rhythms of her day-to-day life have been supplanted by something not entirely or fully anticipated, no matter how carefully she has prepared herself for this moment. She has passed from health into hurting, from wholeness into feeling fragmented. This is a transitional state as the mind struggles with the pain, the body with the invasive process, the psyche with overload. Sleep is often difficult.

My patient first confronts her wounds some twenty-four to seventy-two hours after surgery. It is, for most, a moment of truth and a vital part of the process of inner transformation—the "changing of the mind" that takes place after surgery. If the patient has spent the night—which I recommend after surgeries that require relative immobility, such as abdominoplasties, facelifts, or combined procedures—I will unwrap the bandages and look at the incisions. She will sometimes look as well, but if she seems light-headed or nauseated, I will instruct her to avert her eyes. The incisions are always dotted with blood or bruised during the first days after surgery. Some patients will have trouble looking at them.

My role now is that of a caretaker and guardian, helping the patient reenter the world. As I change the dressing, I will address concerns and give lots of encouragement. If I have performed facial surgery, I tell her to avoid mirrors for the moment and to surround herself only with those who will offer support to aid healing. Before my patient goes home, the nurses will teach her how to empty the blood out of the plastic drain tubes into plastic cups that measure the blood.

I have discovered that patients who will not look at the wounds in the first week after surgery or who refuse to deal with their drains do not heal as well as those who do. Nor do those patients who do not set aside time to recover, who power right back into their lives. Nor do those patients who don't want to talk to other patients about the experience beforehand or see pictures of the scars. By minimizing the depth of their experience—which includes the risk they are undertaking as well as the reality of the scar—they end up minimizing the results. They are less aware of the stories that underlie their choice to have surgery and, for them, the transformation cosmetic surgery offers is more likely to be confined to the surface. Paradoxically, they are both more likely to be dissatisfied with the results of the surgery, on the one hand, and, on the other, most likely to be the women who seek out repeat procedures as a panacea to other problems.

Similarly, patients who try to control the entire process and come in armed with pages of notes and articles—and who try to show me how they want me to perform the surgery—are unlikely to be transformed in any meaningful sense. They are, I believe, unable to surrender to the leap into the unknown that surgery represents; willing surrender is part of what the journey into wholeness requires.

Those who keep their surgery secret—thus denying themselves the privilege and benefit of having witnesses to their experience who can help acknowledge the inner change—will only be transformed on the surface. Their own ambivalence about choosing surgery will also limit the degree to which the experience can change them meaningfully. Finally, women in pursuit of physical perfection who believe that a perfect body or face is a quid pro quo for happiness in life or for getting what they want will not experience real healing. These are the women whose own sense of self is entirely defined by the world's perception of their outer selves and who do not see themselves whole. The inner self and the outer self aren't connected in these women, and truth—essential to healing—is often missing from their discussions of their lives and their reasons for undergoing surgery. I know from experience that surgery will not help them to love themselves more or to perceive themselves as worthy of love.

In marked contrast are the patients who have been most aware of why they have chosen surgery and who have, throughout the process, acknowledged the risks that surgery entails. Their choices have been formed by the need to acknowledge or facilitate a life change or passage, and they will heal more quickly because their choice is embodied and conscious. These are also the women who will acknowledge their wounds as well as their discomfort. And for them, the days and weeks that follow will constitute true transformation.

I have come to realize that the inner transformation that surgery offers depends almost entirely on intention; awareness; informed, conscious decision; and willing submission. The more conscious the choice, the greater potential of true healing.

Why is that?

One patient of mine explained it simply but eloquently in a note she wrote to me some years ago: "If I can see and control my wound, I can heal myself. If I can surrender to being cut, I can surrender to life in the moment without fear." Although the idea of choosing to be wounded may sound strange, willing wounds—those chosen by the patient—are very different in kind from those received by accident, and can be a source of tremendous empowerment precisely because they are chosen. This pattern is most evident in my patients who have undergone previous surgeries because of disease, accident, or other trauma and who have then chosen to undergo cosmetic surgery to propel themselves onto a different life path. The surrender to being cut is, as my patient understood, a willing surrender to living and taking on the risks living fully entails.

One extraordinary woman, a patient I treated several years ago, stands out in this regard. She had been in a devastating car accident at the age of twenty-five, which forever changed the way she looked. Disfigured by injuries and burns, she had undergone thirty-seven separate reconstructive surgeries over the years and had had, in a very basic sense, to invent herself anew. When she came into my private office, I saw her poise first and then took in her face, feature by feature: the still-beautiful eyes and high cheekbones, framed by a network of thick scars around her reconstructed nose and mouth. She'd made no effort to hide or disguise the scars. She had come to me to have her breasts lifted, and she was very clear about what she wanted. I asked her the same question I always ask: "Why now?"

Her answer was simple and direct. She was turning forty. A new relationship seemed to offer new possibilities. She was ready, she felt, to move forward, and from her point of view, having her breasts lifted would signal leaving the accident behind and putting it firmly in the past. For her, choosing surgery also signaled her acceptance of herself and the scars she had not chosen. Not coincidentally, it was also the fifteenth anniversary of her life-changing accident. I came to understand that, after years of submitting to surgery, choosing cosmetic surgery was a gesture of self-articulation and agency. While deciding to lift her breasts might have been a way of asserting her femininity, I also thought that the specific part of her body she'd chosen to alter was meaningful but not all-important. What truly mattered to her was marking the turning point in her life—making her new life trajectory manifest. In her case, the "willing wound"— after submitting to reconstructive surgery thirty-seven times over a fifteen-year period—was indeed a surrender to life and all the possibilities it offers.

Being able to "surrender to life"—with all of its inherent risks— is a key to the process of living fully and consciously and being open to spiritual and psychological transformation. This is complicated terrain, for in order to grow, we must also take leave of the safe and comfortable places in our lives and minds and embark on an entirely new journey. In his book, *Love, Medicine and Miracles,* Dr. Bernie Siegel writes about the spiritual transcendence and enrichment that, paradoxically, can come out of life-threatening illness or crisis. He explains that "to unblock the fountain of love and enter on the path of creative spiritual growth, we must let go of our fears. But this is very hard, particularly when it looks as though we're not going to die tomorrow. When we don't have that time limit, it's often harder to let go."[1] The crisis of illness often frees people to let go of their fears—as they surrender to the unknown—and permits them to learn to love themselves and others. Knowing that we will not live forever, Dr. Siegel notes, puts us into the present with intensity, and allows us to rid ourselves of fears that have held us back in the past. It is then, and only then, that we can embark on the "path of creative spiritual growth."[2]

Like illness, surgery—with its intense physicality, its engagement of the self—can wake us up to the present moment, to our own truth and the truths around us. It also constitutes a surrender or letting go. It forces us to acknowledge the truth of inhabiting our impermanent bodies in the present. It helps us to accept both our vulnerability and mortality as well as our need for the help of others; in that sense, it can also free us of the fear of loss and death. Its inherent violence—the piercing of the skin, the outer armor of the self—forces a disintegration of the self, fragmented by pain, which in turn swings open a door to reintegration and growth, similar in kind to the growth experienced by the individual in a rite of passage. It is a modern form of what Joseph Campbell called the rite of passage's "severe exercise of severance." The recovery from surgery in this context, with a conscious and embodied patient, becomes an act of community as well, illuminating the ties to those around us, on whom we depend for help and support during this time.

While it seems paradoxical that willing fragmentation is the key to a journey into wholeness—the model proposed by the rite of passage—it doesn't appear that inner transformation in human beings can take place without significant initial disruption, pain, and a leaving behind of parts of the self, whether we call them "necessary losses" as Judith Viorst did or stages in an initiatory process. To rebuild the self, the older self must first be taken down with force. Not surprisingly, contemporary strategies to help the individual achieve inner change—such as psychotherapy—also follow the same pattern as ritual initiation.

As Robert L. Moore has pointed out, all psychotherapeutic strategies have much in common with initiatory stages. Just as the initiate must submit to the ritual process, so, too, the patient must submit to the therapeutic process, willingly committing time and money. Just as the initiate moves out of familiar surroundings into transformative space, so, too, the patient enters into the therapist's office, which operates by rules very different from those in the outside world. The therapist's office is the space where that which is hidden can be brought out into the open, where the unsaid can be said, where fears can be faced safely. Finally, like the elder in a rite of passage, the therapist enacts a drama with the patient that facilitates a confrontation with the feelings and events that have prevented the patient from moving on in his or her life. During this confrontation, the patient's defenses are breached and the false or older self disintegrates under pressure, which allows the true self to emerge.[3]

The overall pattern remains the same: Growth requires wounding, disintegration, or loss so that wholeness can follow. Because our society's take on cosmetic surgery confines it to the surface and tends to minimize the wounding the patient undergoes, the way in which even elective surgery re-creates the physical and psychological conditions necessary for inner growth has been ignored.

But, nonetheless, researchers studying how body image changes after cosmetic surgery have focused on how the foundation for cognitive change is perceptual change—what the patient sees in the mirror—and how she "feels" those changes. They've noted that having the body or body part feel "different"—even if the sensation is negative, such as the loss of nipple sensation after breast reduction—facilitates cognitive change. The fact of feeling is enough to change the patient's thinking.[4]

Most fascinating—though not surprising from my point of view—is their discussion of pain and psychological distress after cosmetic surgery. Researchers observed that patients who had the most marked negative emotional reactions in the postoperative period would actually experience the most positive emotional outcomes in the long term. Questioning why this happened, the authors ventured that this clinical phenomenon might be related to theories of psychological change that propose that change must always be preceded by a period of disruption "before reorganization and lasting benefit can take place."[5]

I believe that the physical, psychological, emotional, and social disruption surgery produces allows it to become a pathway to a new future for the individual.

Surgery as a Portal

Both my own stories and those of many of my patients, each of whom related their surgery to a crisis or turning point in their lives, permitted me to see surgery as a possible portal to true transformation. It became clear that certain periods of upheaval in our lives—times of psychological unrest when the mere forward motion of day-to-day life doesn't carry us far enough—in fact could become springboard moments for change, allowing us to wrest control and take charge of our own stories. For many of us, this reformulation of the self will include changing the way we look. Thus, even though our culture tends to see choosing cosmetic surgery as an act of self-hatred, it is often an act of self-love.

Something in our human nature seems to require that we mark those internal changes ritualistically, creating a visible marker that reminds us of our new story. At a time of crisis or after a landmark event, we redecorate our homes, move, or start over in some other symbolic way. For more profound inner changes, we turn to our bodies to tell our new stories. These markers can be impermanent, such as by coloring or cutting our hair, or changing our style, or they can be permanent, such as by getting a piercing or a tattoo, or modifying the body through surgery. For some women, the more important the life change, the greater the need for permanent marking. Sometimes the marker declares the change already made, as in the case of patients who have lost tremendous amounts of weight through serious dieting and exercise and then decide to have surgery to mark the conclusion of the journey. Other times, having the surgery is a declaration of a new stage of life. I have had many patients who have followed their surgeries with life-changing decisions such as leaving a long-term marriage or switching careers, just as I have seen survivors of illness do.

I learned many years ago that the acquisition of the marker—the scar left behind by the surgery, the physical change wrought by the surgery or by exercise and diet—gives the inner change an external reality. This was brought home by the observation of a patient who confided that she envied a woman who had been scarred by illness. Baffled, I asked her why. The scar was something, she explained, that testified to the woman's suffering and made it palpable and real. She, on the other hand, doubted the memory of her own emotional experience because it had no physical manifestation.

Interior emotional changes—wrought by experiences such as birth, death, loss, or change in an important relationship—are also understood by patients as needing to be shown to the world in physical form. One patient wrote me after surgery, expressing her appreciation for "an external expression of a new beginning made from the clay of the past. . . . There are many opportunities along the way to make a new choice, to shed skin, to regenerate into that which most closely resembles our inner essence and true nature." Bringing the inner and outer selves into alignment is a persistent theme in many of my patients' narratives of self.

I have had many patients who want to have scars left by traumatic events removed; I tell them that while the scar cannot be removed, it can be transformed into something they choose. In this way, the old scar becomes a "willing wound" and permits the patient to recast the past into a new context. While, from a surgical point of view, transforming a scar is technically easy, navigating the emotional terrain associated with the scar is usually complicated. One woman had had Hodgkin's disease as a child and had undergone mantle radiation to her chest area and, as a result, had underdeveloped breasts. By choosing augmentation, she moved from seeing herself as a "sickly child"—the sense of self formed by her illness—to being a healthy and fit adult. She went on to run a triathlon.

Many women choose abdominoplasty to transform the cesarian scars left behind by a disappointing or disruptive experience of childbirth or pregnancy. This decision is often connected symbolically to the patient's own identity as a mother as well as to the stories of her daughterhood and her own mother. There was the woman who had given birth to her daughter under extremely traumatic circumstances, undergoing a caesarean section without adequate anesthesia. When she turned forty-five—which was one year older than her mother had been when she died—she chose to have an abdominoplasty to change the association of trauma and suffering with the birth, as well as to transform the scar left behind. Symbolically, she said good-bye to the self who mourned her mother as well as to the self who had suffered during birth. The surgery permitted her to welcome in a new self who found new joy in motherhood.

These are instances in which, by surgically altering the storied part of the body, the patient is able to recast both the story of the body part and her larger inner narrative as well. This doesn't deny that some women will pursue cosmetic surgery—actually, more likely multiple cosmetic surgeries—*instead* of making the change they need to. I think that these women look to surgery as a magic pill or an event that will miraculously catapult them into a transformed existence, but without inner work, it simply doesn't happen.

Sometimes, though, the details belie the process that is going on beneath the surface. I had one patient who came in in the wake of discovering her husband's affair with a much younger woman. She had already begun to mark her body with tattoos and now wanted a facelift. The facelift was a technical success but the marital relationship continued to deteriorate. The husband moved out, though they stayed married, and she went on to have breast implants and an abdominoplasty. I'm usually leery of performing multiple cosmetic procedures on a single patient but, as it happens, she had been referred by a colleague with good judgment about motivation and character. As the patient approached her third surgery with the help of ongoing therapy and the support of her church, she finally decided to leave her husband. She not only left him and changed careers, but was fully supported by her children both in her decision to have the last surgery and to divorce their father. While the conventional way of looking at her story would be to understand her surgeries as a way of pleasing her husband or competing with a younger rival in the mode of a made-for-television movie, I believe something else also took place. Surgery represented the experience she needed to change her mind, to jump-start her into action, so that she could do what she needed to do. It may have given her the courage to take on the risk of changing her life. I saw her not long ago and she was radiant and happy and, in addition to a new career, has a new and loving relationship.

While some people seem to be capable of effecting changes in their lives with ease, I have come to appreciate that others require drastic circumstances to awaken and redirect themselves. Sometimes illness, accident, or personal catastrophe—such as the death of a loved one—will set the stage for a new life story and give individuals who have long known that they need to change their lives the impetus to do so. As a physician, I am hardly alone in making this observation. As Dean Ornish has noted, writing of his work with heart patients and the lifestyles that underlie disease, "Most of us are deeply attached to our belief systems and are resistant to change. However, when we are in pain, the status quo becomes less desirable. There is an opportunity for real change."[6] For one of my patients, long overweight, the death of his mother signaled the beginning of a three-year journey to transform his body and his sense of self. He lost some one hundred twenty pounds and has now undergone surgery to remove excess skin on his fiftieth birthday. He explained both simply and eloquently: "I have new tools and intuition to live life from the inside out, rather than from outside in."

The symbolism of choosing surgery can be astonishing both in its power and meaning. One patient was an identical twin who had lived a life very much in tandem with her sister. They were married within a year of each other, each had five children within a year or so of each other, and each had had the experience of losing a child.

My patient came in wanting a breast lift shortly after her sister had been treated for aggressive breast cancer and had a mastectomy and reconstruction. Among the reasons she chose to have surgery was a symbolic one so that her life path could continue to converge with her sister's.

Changing the Body, Changing the Mind

While elective surgery can be a celebration or marking of a change already made—such as in a career or a relationship—or a commemoration of an important event, it can equally be a catalyst. Surgery is simultaneously a life interruption as well as a life transition, which creates both a "before" and an "after" that is real and undeniable. It suspends the patient's "present" and anticipates an immediate future, which will require stamina and fortitude. Science confirms what I have seen in my patients: that undergoing surgery may bring with it a veritable flood of positive energy, which can yield a quantum leap in spiritual and emotional growth. It changes the patient in ways that go beyond the physical because the process of choosing the surgery, preparing for it, undergoing it, and recovering from it become part of the patient's bank of life experiences that redefine the self.

While science once held that the pathways of the brain, governing how we think and remember, became fixed as we age, the research of the last two decades has shown that throughout our adulthood our brains change and adjust as we acquire new knowledge and create new memories. We now know that experience literally changes how the neural circuits in our brains are organized and work, a phenomenon referred to as "brain plasticity." Learning and experience modify the internal structure of the neurons as well as increase the number of synapses between them. It's not just classroom learning or an emotional event that alters those neural patterns, but physical experiences such as accidents, illness, and surgery. The connection between the mind and the body is both simple and complicated at once and takes place on different levels of awareness or consciousness.

On the simplest level, as Dr. Herbert Benson points out in his book *Timeless Healing*, the brain is "ever-changing." As he says, "Every new experience, every new fact entered into your brain changes its configuration and your awareness of who you were, who you are, and who you will be. Because of the brain's intrinsic malleability, you have the ability to literally 'change your mind.'" As he notes, even the act of reading forges new connections in the brain, whether you are reading his book or mine or any other.[7] In this sense, the power of transformation is literally built into the basic structure of the human organism, as is the mechanism by which we redefine the meaning of events and interactions in our lives.

On a more complex level, the entity we call the "self" is also plastic and is modified in large ways and small as both the body and the brain respond to the stimulus of experience. The remodeling that takes place on a neural level is echoed in our own evolving identity. The self—as each of us would readily acknowledge—is, on the one hand, an apparently stable entity, which we can describe and identify by characteristic responses and traits, likes and dislikes. We are able to say that something isn't "me" or that someone isn't "for us" precisely because of those aspects of the self, familiar and recognizable. On the other hand, we also understand that our personal narratives—how we tell our stories and describe ourselves—shift at different times in our lives. Our sense of self is both stable and fluid at once. We may describe ourselves as malleable and easily influenced during one period of our lives, and as hard-nosed and resolute during another, without thinking that these contradictions point to anything other than a unified "self."

What permits us to form a cogent and consistent sense of self is what Antonio Damasio has called "autobiographical memory." Autobiographical memory is made up of personal traits and all of our experiences in life, large and small. A grab bag of things that make the self, those experiences range, as he notes, "from simple to complex, from benign to dangerous, involving anything from trivial preferences to ethical principles."[8]

This autobiographical memory is subject to constant remodeling over time and is reshaped by experiences in the present and our understanding of past experience. In addition, the autobiographical self is rewritten and reshaped by our anticipation of the future.[9]

With that idea in mind, considering cosmetic surgery as something that affects "only" the surface belies what science knows about the interconnection of the brain, the body, and that entity we call the self. Instead, when we consider choosing cosmetic surgery, we need to think about it as a potential catalyst that may not only change how we think about ourselves in the future but may also offer us the opportunity to reimagine the past. It is an event that can, in fact, substantially revise how we see all the different elements of the autobiographical self.

Surgery has this extraordinary potential precisely because it engages and involves the mind and the body at once and forcibly moves us from one state of being (intact and connected) to another (wounded and separate). The scar it leaves marks the territory of where we have been and separates it from where we are going. The experience of surrendering to the surgical process as well as recovering from it allows us to transform not just the outer layer of our bodies but the inner strata of our storied selves.

Conscious Process

Plastic surgeons aren't psychologists or therapists, but given the profound connection between the outer body and inner self, it might be argued that they should be. As the connection between surgery and the rituals that facilitated and celebrated life passages became clearer to me, I saw that supporting the patient's awareness was key to making the surgery as successful as it could be, and I began to incorporate strategies to make that possible.

The first stage of making the surgical process conscious begins with meeting the patient to identify the new physical form she seeks. I don't use computer imaging because I believe it often offers a promise that the surgeon can't fulfill and makes it seem as though the outcome of the surgery is guaranteed in ways it cannot be. Computer imaging doesn't account for the real variations from patient to patient, surgery to surgery, in healing, bleeding, and scarring, because general nutrition and health affect healing in ways that are known and unknown. Scars, while more hidden in certain surgeries (facelifts, for example), are an inevitable part of the process. Despite what you may have read about "scarless surgery" or "noninvasive skin tightening," my profession hasn't succeeded in realizing either of these—not yet, at least. Bringing the inner image into the real world includes, of necessity, understanding that the more loose skin there is, the more scarring there will be. It's important that the patient keep in mind the risk/benefit ratio when we discuss contour and tightness.

We look at photographs of previous patients to see what most resembles her mental image of her physical transformation. The act of choosing the photograph enables the patient to move the desired physical result from her imagination into the real world so that we can discuss it directly and in detail.

At this point, I can assess whether the patient's desires are realistic because managing expectations—what surgery can and can't accomplish—is central to the process. In my own experience, the technical success of any surgery as seen by the doctor is, in fact, less important than the patient's internal assessment of the change she has experienced, very little of which actually depends on what she sees in the mirror. Apparently, I am not alone; an article in the *New York Times* about "do over" surgery (that is, cosmetic surgery performed by one doctor and "redone" by another), notes that "what looks good" is highly subjective, and as one doctor put it, expected outcomes are "negotiated" between doctor and patient.[10] Research done by Thomas Pruzinsky and Milton T. Edgerton posits that patient satisfaction with surgical results has three components: surgical, psychological, and social. Surgical expectations focus solely on appearance, while psychological expectations have much to do with the benefits to feelings of self-worth, improvement of body image, and the quality of life patients hope surgery will offer them. The social expectations focus on social interactions and how a changed appearance will improve them.[11] It's clear that keeping these expectations realistic will have much to do with whether the patient perceives the surgery as "successful" on all three levels.

Women seeking breast reduction or augmentation look at a book filled with images of breasts in all shapes and sizes. I explain the variations in cleavage, nipple position, and the like, and go into details about the possible loss of sensation and scarring. For rhinoplasty, I will draw on a photograph of the patient in her presence after she's brought in pictures of noses she likes. At this point, I will tell her if I can accomplish what she's seeking. Each part of the nose—the tip, the bridge, the projection, and the nasolabial angle—is discussed in detail. For a patient seeking a facelift, I will ask what bothers her most about her face as it is now and what she would like to change. Sometimes I will have her bring in photographs taken when she was younger. I will explain in detail what I can—and can't—accomplish. I've learned that patients who bring in photos taken within the last decade have more reasonable expectations than those who bring in pictures that are twenty years old. This exercise is a good litmus test both for patient satisfaction or dissatisfaction postoperatively, as well as helping to expose her expectations about the surgery.

The discussion brings the patient's mental image into the real world and, in addition, lets me listen to some of her internal narrative. Since all parts of the body are storied, this discussion gives me some access to the narrative threads that connect the body part she intends to change to her sense of herself now and in the future. Every internal picture of a physical feature—nose, breasts, buttocks, face—is highly subjective and, as we've already seen, may have very little to do with the "reality" glimpsed in a mirror. Instead, the body part is tied to a highly symbolic interior narrative that defines the present self and that, once altered by surgery, will redefine the self. How and to what degree the self is redefined depends on many factors, only one of which is the technical success of the surgery itself.

A patient may also connect her body part symbolically or literally to emotional states or definitions of self. One woman described how, after her divorce, she felt enormous conflict between her role as the single mother of a daughter and her reawakened sexual self. While she had loved being a full-time mother when her daughter was young, she felt increasingly conflicted as she approached the age of forty. She was no longer sure that she wanted, as she put it, to sacrifice herself completely to her child, and the guilt she felt when dating and socializing took her away from her child only exacerbated her sense of crisis. She longed to reconcile the split she felt as a mother and a sexual being. Not surprisingly, the part of her body that made her unhappy was her belly—which was left with extra skin, stretch marks, fat and scars from her C-section, all resistant to exercise and diet. She saw changing her belly through surgery as a way to heal the rift within her, and decided to have the surgery on a date right before her own fortieth birthday and her daughter's fourteenth. Her daughter's age was important because fourteen had marked her own coming of age, a time she associated with growth and connection and independence. She saw forty as a landmark age for herself, and thought that choosing surgery symbolized a commitment to put her own needs on the table along with her child's. It did not surprise me that the date of her surgery coincided with both her and her child's life transitions.

Patients often connect the symbolic nature of the transformation to real-world results. While I try to dissuade patients from making this connection literally—cosmetic surgery will not necessarily facilitate making more money or getting a new job or finding the right lover—it may well energize or empower them sufficiently to meet their own goals. One woman, not a patient of mine as it happens, had a facelift in her late forties. Long divorced, she'd had spectacular success in the business world for some fifteen years but, by her own lights, was beginning to feel and look tired. When asked if the surgery had transformed more than the surface, she grimaced, saying that the recovery had been much harder and more painful than she had anticipated. Then she smiled and went on to tell the story of how, a year after the surgery, she met and married the man she is happily married to today. And how, in her mid-fifties, she went back to school, earned a Ph.D., and started a new career. When asked if the surgery had been a catalyst for the beginning of a new life journey, she simply said, "I don't know exactly. But I do know that everything changed after I had it."

I would say instead that the surgery woke her up to the moment and helped her gather up the strength to make the other necessary changes in her life.

"Unconscious" Decisions and Surgery

While patients who aren't in touch with their inner stories and who deny the import of surgery are unlikely to be transformed in any real way, others who ignore the signals sent by either their body or their psyche may actually be at risk. I often recommend that a patient postpone surgery if her consultation reveals that she is in the middle of a life transition such as caring for someone who is ill or going through a divorce, or a particularly stressful situation, such as changing jobs or moving. One patient had scheduled a breast reduction and, two weeks before the surgery, developed palpitations and shortness of breath. Her internist suggested that it was anxiety, but she denied she was nervous about her surgery, saying that she had all her affairs in order, including her will. That comment raised a red flag for me, and I subsequently learned that she was caring for her mother, who was terminally ill. I postponed the surgery. I felt that her surgery was, in some sense, a distraction from her present situation, and while choosing surgery under those circumstances might still be an act of self-assertion, her symptoms made it clear that her mind and her body were not at one.

While there are practical reasons not to have surgery at a time of high stress or life transition—such as when there are problems with having enough support or being able to commit fully to the recovery—practicality isn't the only concern. The psychological commitment to the surgical process and the recovery must be complete, and the mind and the body must be in sync. Because surgery is a stressor, how emotionally charged a woman's life is at any given point should be part of the decision on whether to go forward with it. An extreme example is the case I was asked to review some time ago, of a woman who died of postoperative complications. Recently widowed, the woman had scheduled relatively minor cosmetic surgery. At the very last minute, she decided to have more extensive surgery; the surgeon did not inquire into her emotional state, though the nurses in the office remembered her as very sad and nervous. She had, apparently, been bowled over by grief and depression with no support, and had wanted to move on with her life. It wasn't to be.

There are other situations in which patients should be either encouraged to postpone surgery or discouraged from having it at all. Some women are single- mindedly focused on a physical characteristic, so much so that they ignore what is really going on in their lives. I had a patient who fixated on her nose, though from an "objective" point of view, there was nothing observably wrong with it. It took several consultations for me to hear the real, if buried, expectations she had for surgery—that a "new" nose would land her a modeling career and fix her relationship with her lover. In the most profound sense, her expectations could not be met—and I didn't operate on her. There are other potential patients who need to be discouraged from proceeding with surgery. The woman who uses surgery to remain a victim is likely to have a higher rate of complication. So is the patient who denies that the body part she wishes to change has a story other than its physical manifestation, and the woman who projects her anxiety onto the results of a previous surgery, seeking correction after correction without looking at why she had the surgery initially.

Some women will intuitively understand when the time is right for their surgery. I performed a facelift on a woman not long ago who admitted she had wanted one for close to a decade, and her case is the perfect example of conscious choice. The last eight or so years of her life had been extremely trying; her husband had been stricken with cancer and died slowly and painfully. During that time, she had thought of having a facelift. She hadn't pursued it, she said, because it seemed "too vain" and "self-centered" in the context of life as it was then. Then her husband died and she grieved terribly and alone for three years. She still thought about a facelift but, in her isolation, the time still didn't feel right. Then she reunited with a man she'd dated in high school and her life took a totally new turn. She came to see me a year after they were married, when the time was finally right. "Why now?" I asked. "I never thought I'd smile again," she said, "and now I'm with a man who makes me laugh. I want my face to show the difference."

When Surgery Is a Substitute

Just as there are women who will turn to substitute behaviors such as disordered eating during a life crisis, so, too, there are women who turn to cosmetic surgery as a substitute. Women in midlife who are overwhelmed by or unable to deal with the crises of the transition—a stalled career, a house without children, a floundering marriage—and choose instead to focus on restoring their youth through surgery as a way of avoiding the larger, more difficult issues, are one such group.

Surgery in this circumstance becomes a way of distracting the self and denying the issues at hand, and many such women will seek out repeat procedures for precisely this reason.

I've noticed that patients who use cosmetic surgery as a tactic of avoidance will often suffer from minor depression after their procedure, particularly after a facelift. Because they've chosen the procedure not to mark a life passage but to deny it, they are unlikely to benefit from the transformative potential of the surgery itself. Their depression will usually lift when they are validated by the outside world on the results of the surgery, which might be something as simple as someone saying they look years younger.

In all of these cases, transformation will be limited to the surface changes wrought by the surgeon.

As the connection between surgery and rites of passage became clear to me, I began to appreciate that the more conscious the decision to undergo a procedure was, the better the results. It was at this time that I fully recognized why my own second procedure—the liposuction—had been problematic. Rather than an act of self-love, it was a substitute for dealing with ambivalences about myself and my relationship to my ex-husband. In retrospect, I wished that someone had simply asked me, "Why are you doing this now?" or "Why does this part of your body bother you?" in an insistent enough voice so that I might have been required to answer.

I also came to see that women who decide to undergo cosmetic surgery needed to explore the storied aspects of their bodies, to get in touch with the personal symbolism of the part of their bodies they have decided to alter, and to put their decision into the context of their lives. By doing all of these things, they could avail themselves of the opportunity to transform themselves both inside and out.

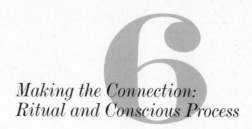

Making the Connection:
Ritual and Conscious Process

When I was in training as a young surgeon on the cardiac ward, I had a very clear idea of what constituted "being alive." It was definable, measurable, even visible on the monitors in front of me. Now, all these years later, I realize that life is defined more subtly and with more difficulty. What about the force of purpose—the essence of being human—without which the heart is no more than a muscle pumping blood? Alternatively, what about the definition of life when the heart beats, the oxygen flows through the tissues, but the activity of the brain is blunted or absent?

In the same way, how I understood the meaning of healing—the act of making whole—began to shift. Whatever insight I garnered, I gained piecemeal, case by case. I remember the young woman who was rushed into the hospital after a drug overdose; the team "saved" her with a liver transplant that she neither asked for nor consented to. After her body "healed," she was released back into the same spiritless, purposeless world from which she had tumbled into the emergency room, without friends or family or support. Her body restored but her spirit still lacerated, she attempted suicide again. We'd done nothing to change the stories that propelled her forward or defined her self. We hadn't sutured her soul.

If I have learned anything, it is that the relationship of the body and the mind or spirit—in sickness or wholeness—is tightly choreographed, an inextricable partnership. Neither illness nor health is ever "all in the body" or "all in the mind." Body and mind are interwoven in ways we are only beginning to understand through the reaches of Western scientific inquiry; our muscles and tissues hold memories stored way too deep for our waking conscious minds to retrieve. Every emotion, thought, and event we've experienced through the mind is written on our bodies somewhere—in an alphabet of neural pathways, created by the release of hormones. In the same way, the experiences of our bodies—confrontations with danger, the exertion of a marathon run, the engagement of rituals, the pleasure of lovemaking, the pain of a wound—reach the mind and change the neural pathways in the brain, and thus the stories and the architecture of the self. The truth of the dyad of mind and body has long been known in Eastern traditions, though largely forgotten or ignored until recently in the West.

Healing must always involve both the body and the spirit. There is no true transformation unless the two are fully engaged in the effort. All change occurs through the window of the body; it isn't possible to undergo transformation simply by thinking about it or by conceiving it. It must be experienced through the body in a literal way.

Perhaps the greatest cost of our wrongheaded, if persistent, belief in the mind/body split has been our refusal to see this single truth. Instead, we insist that the need to change the body radically is always motivated by superficiality, vanity, or succumbing to cultural pressure. Our belief in the superiority of the mind encourages us to ignore what our bodies tell us, and to distrust the signals our bodies send us. We underestimate the importance of what we have experienced in and through our bodies and how it connects to how we feel about ourselves in the broadest sense. We look away from the stories our bodies tell us, and discount them as a source of wisdom and growth. The only context in which we understand pain—whether it is experienced physically through the body or psychologically through the mind—is as something to be avoided or "overcome," instead of a potential source of energy to be harnessed in order to change the stories of the self.

Our attitude toward pain affects both the individual and the culture as a whole. We are uncomfortable even as witnesses to another human being's pain, and shy away from situations that require us to be present as witnesses. As Rachel Naomi Remen has remarked, "We've been taught since childhood that pain is 'poor form' and often to react to it as if it is a breach of good manners. In other cultures, pain and loss are not as lonely."[1] As a result, we paper over pain instead of confronting it and lose, in the process, the understanding that growth is always preceded by pain. When we are physically healthy, transformation depends on psychological and emotional sacrifice—giving up cherished needs and convictions—in order to open up to the new. The pain we feel is emotional and psychological in nature, although it is often stored in the body or integrated into how we experience our bodies as well.

Similarly, our belief in the mind-body split deprives us of understanding physical pain as a possible window to spiritual growth. Our resistance to pain often becomes a rejection of experience, and it's been suggested, from both a psychological and spiritual point of view, that by resisting pain, we only increase our suffering. Spiritual teachers such as Thich Nhat Hanh amplify this thought by distinguishing between pain and suffering. Suffering, he writes, "is the psychological amplification of pain through resistance." Pain, on the other hand, "can be converted breath by breath, into an awakening chime to mindfulness." Because pain brings us into the present with force and intensity, it opens the door to greater awareness.

For most of my patients, the surgical process is part of a journey toward spiritual integrity that, along the way, includes an acceptance of pain as well as the process of healing. By confronting and listening to their bodies' stories, they are able to rewrite them through surgery with a sense of agency and empowerment. Paradoxical as it may sound, they discover that changing their bodies not only symbolizes their inner transformation but affirms and facilitates it. The ritualistic nature of surgery accomplishes this in part, but after years in practice, I realized that the experience of transformation can be intensified and bolstered by other rituals that underscore and support the symbolism of the transformation surgery represents.

To that end, five years ago I began offering my patients a more conscious way of approaching surgery, by working with ritualists, psychotherapists, and others in the healing professions. While we can't literally imitate the way rites of passage worked in older societies—sequestering the individual for months, for example, or calling up his or her elders to bear witness—we *can* work with the patient's inner landscape to help create rituals that will help him or her to make the whole surgical process more fully conscious and embodied. In this way, healing after surgery includes both the body and spirit, and can move the individual to a new level of wholeness.

The rituals we help the patient create are based on time-honored models but are tailored to each individual so that she can best express her own inner story and passage. The ritual preparations include keeping a dream journal; building an altar to clarify her intentions and give them physical form; practicing meditation; and creating prayers and words to accompany the surgery. To the extent that we can, we encourage the patient to seek the active involvement of friends, family, and other loved ones.

How Ritual Works

The purpose of ritual is to make conscious what is beneath the surface in the mind of the individual and the community. It also makes the ordinary sacred, by raising the awareness of the meaning and energy involved in simple acts. All rituals seek to have the individual experience and act through symbol, sight, sound, and feeling.

More than ever, ritual is a necessary corrective to the spiritual vacuum most of us experience, whether we are at a moment of life transition or not. Our daily lives—rushed and impatient—may appear on the surface to be engaged, but in reality, our busyness may be nothing more than a distraction from what really feeds our spirits. With so much of our energy and attention directed at and absorbed in the small details—getting the kids off to school and going to work, running our errands, making time for the gym, sitting down to a meal that is sandwiched between other activities—we risk losing connection to the underlying rhythms of what matters in the long run and to the turning points or crises in our lives. We start living on autopilot, ignoring the signs and signals that we have reached a crossroad. This state is familiar to most of us from one period of our lives or another: a time when we are so caught up in the act of living that we forget the meaning of life and find ourselves sleepwalking through it. It is what the existential philosopher Heidegger called a state of "forgetfulness of being."

In contrast there is mindfulness of being—the moment at which we are fully self-aware and conscious of the power innate in being the composers of our own lives. Mindfulness is especially important at times of passage when we need all the strength we can muster to navigate the turbulence the transition creates. Conversely, it is "forgetfulness of being" that can lead women to deny the passage at hand or to engage in substitute behavior. Ritual can increase this sense of mindfulness through symbolic action.

How this works is both subtle and powerful, for ritual uses symbolic gestures to invoke, address, and even manipulate us through feeling and sensation. We disconnect from the "ordinary" world, the distraction of details, and the workings of rational thought, and connect to a different kind of perception through the use of pattern and repetition. Rituals are perceived through the senses—through sound, sight, and touch—and are felt rather than analyzed; we respond to them through the right side of our brains, not the left. Rituals answer the larger questions of purpose—Why are we here? What do we want from our lives?—not with explanatory sentences but with the evocation of the larger patterns that animate our lives.

One ritual our culture continues to honor—the wedding ceremony—has lost much of its gravitas but still illuminates the general structure and function of ritual. An assembly is gathered, most usually in a place considered sacred or set apart, to witness the life passage of two individuals. Details—special garments, decorations, music, flowers—set the moment apart from the ordinary and underscore its import. The joining of the individuals is symbolically enacted through gestures—the exchange of repeated vows; the reading of sacred or special texts; the exchange of rings; the kiss, which symbolizes their spiritual and sexual union. A marriage license, as Tom Driver notes, "doesn't create a marriage but simply gives permission for a wedding ceremony to take place." It is the ceremony, civil or religious, short or long, that brings the marriage into being. Thus, Driver writes, "rites of passage are performed not simply to *mark* transitions but to *effect* them."[2]

In its formalized gestures, its repetition, its exaggeration, its symbolism, and its dramatic flourishes, ritual both distinguishes the transformative event from everyday life and helps bring it into being. The use of ritual before the surgery has, for some of my patients, had similar results, and has given the experience of surgery a spiritual dimension that has considerably enriched their lives. I have seen it in the operating room as well because when ritual is enacted, all those who participate and all those who witness are engaged and moved in new and different ways.

With a little bit of effort, any woman who has decided to undergo cosmetic surgery can adapt what we do in my practice to her own circumstances.

Laying the Groundwork

Once a patient has decided to undergo what I call "transformational surgery," a counselor begins with a two-hour session that is intended to be a spiritual and psychological journey of self-exploration. The patient is encouraged to look beyond the surface in order to gain a better understanding of herself in mind, body, and spirit. She begins to explore the stories of her body with a new kind of awareness so that she can understand fully why she has sought out surgery. Some of these stories will be less consciously understood than others. We also focus on life passages or significant events in the patient's life to understand the decision to pursue surgery in all of its aspects. At the end, we will work closely with her to create rituals specifically for her surgery.

Among the questions our counselors ask are:

Are You Willing to Look Beneath the Surface and Explore Your Deeper Feelings About the Surgery You've Chosen?

This question begins the process of opening up the body "story" and its connection to the decision to have surgery. Most patients experience a sense of discovery as they explore their own personal symbolism anew. We encourage patients to imagine a dialogue with the part of the body they intend to have changed so as to move past the obvious—"I want bigger breasts"—to the more profound—"I connect my small breasts with my inability to nurture" or "I connect bigger breasts with the ability to take care of others and thus take better care of myself"—and to bring up all the associations, positive and negative, they have with that part of their body and why.

It's not uncommon for a patient to gain new understanding of relationships and events that have contributed to her body narrative. Through counseling, one woman realized that her surgery, body contouring, constituted the completion of a journey to create what she called a new "opening" of her life. She had recently lost over sixty pounds after a lifetime of obesity and gotten fit; she had also forged new connections with a half brother and half sister she never knew she had. As she put it, her extra flesh had covered her for many years; now she was grateful and relieved to finally be "revealed."

Other patients have discovered close connections between their decision to have surgery and other stories in their lives, which they had thought were unrelated. One woman—still beautiful and youthful looking at forty-five—came to me for a facelift after having undergone other procedures elsewhere. A mother of three, she'd been married to a very successful financial analyst for some twenty years, and lived a comfortable life as a stay-at-home mother. Given her history of multiple procedures, I refused to do the surgery unless she participated in the transformational counseling. We asked her to begin keeping a dream journal, a wholly new experience for her. Within a matter of weeks, she came in without an appointment, crying inconsolably. She confessed that while her marriage was still satisfying in many ways—she and her husband had shared many experiences and he was kind and loving—he had stopped sleeping with her years before and she'd sought refuge in an affair. She was terribly afraid her husband would somehow discover her journal and find out about the affair. The process of confronting her story forced her to realize that she had to get honest with herself. She postponed her surgery at that time and she and her husband went into counseling together. Later she returned for surgery, ready to experience her transformation fully, determined to live honestly and fully. Her previous efforts to change her face—the image she projected to the world—were substitutes for other actions she needed to take, but until she could face her true demons, her surgery could never be transformative.

We often encourage artistically inclined patients to create visual representations of themselves before surgery, in drawings or by using sculpting material. These images of their bodies can be realistic or symbolic, and may show the whole self or just the body part they want to change. Later we have them create images representative of themselves after surgery. This ritual enactment is often highly symbolic, since the portrait of the "before" self usually reveals the "storied" body as the patient imagines it to be perceived in the outside world. More than one patient has literally destroyed the "before" image as an act of closure or letting go.

Depicting the postsurgical body is almost always emotional as well; my patients report that they learn to be at peace with themselves during the process, in part because they have been relieved of the burden of denying their body's story. Drawing or sculpting the postsurgical body is also a powerful exercise because it is a concrete manifestation of dreams and desires; putting those dreams into dimensional form is a symbolic act of agency.

Since all the parts of the body have culturally-inherited, traditional symbolism attached to them, it's not unusual for a patient to discover associations he or she hadn't fully been conscious of before. For women, the breasts and the belly are perhaps two of the most symbolically laden parts of the body, and we have found it helpful to use archetypes contained in myths and stories to explore their meanings more fully. The breast—which is thought of as highly sexualized in our culture—was in other cultures the primary emblem of energy and the life-giving force, as well as all potentiality. The great Egyptian goddess Isis, for example, was understood to have created the Milky Way from her breasts. Similarly, the eye was not just the organ of visual perception but of intellectual and spiritual vision; the lidless open eye was symbolic of enlightenment. By exploring the mythic and linguistic symbolism of the part of the body the patient has decided to change, we can help her put her personal story into a larger context of meaning.

What Made You Decide to Have the Surgery *Now*?

This question is an expansion of the question I ask each patient— "Why now?"—and encourages her to put her decision into a larger context and to explore the motivations that may underlie the choice.

A discussion of life passages and transitions, as well as significant events, is always central to this question, as is the symbolic connection between the part of the body the patient has decided to alter and the life transition she has experienced.

The unfolding of the self is never random; all growth and change happen when the timing is right. Understanding the timing of the decision to undergo surgery as simply a matter of convenience—because "the situation at work is under control" or "my schedule is light" or "my kids are away"—is to ignore or miss the significance of the decision within the context of the patient's life. Similarly, when a patient tells me she is moving ahead because "now I can afford it," I remind her that she has made a conscious decision to spend the money on surgery rather than on something else.

This isn't to say, though, that money—or who pays for the surgery—isn't important. For many of my patients, putting aside the money for the surgery or saving for it is an important part of their sense of agency, as well as their decision-making process. Conversely, patients who have their surgery paid for by others often do not experience internal change. This has important implications for those who receive cosmetic surgery as a gift as if it were just another commodity in a consumer society, a trend with growing popularity reported in the *New York Times* at the end of 2005.[3] This trend contributes to the belief that cosmetic surgery isn't "real" surgery, on the one hand, and, on the other, is likely to leave the patient without any sense of agency. It is also likely to result in surgeries that yield only superficial results. Surgery is something you need to choose for and by yourself.

Sometimes making the connection between the conscious and unconscious intentions is complicated. One woman, after losing eighty pounds and getting herself into top physical shape—cycling and running for the first time in her life—came in seeking an eye lift when the last of her three children left home for college. At the age of fifty-eight, she'd been left with a great deal of loose skin on her body due to her weight loss late in life, as well as some sagging in her face about which she seemed unconcerned; her focus was exclusively on her eyes, which, while slightly hooded, might not have bothered another person. Through counseling, we discovered that when her own mother had experienced the empty nest, she became bitter and depressed, and no longer felt she had a role in life. She refused all offers of help, and died a few years later, unhappy and unfulfilled. For this patient, her mother's narrowed eyes symbolized withdrawal from love and affection, and when she looked at her own face in the mirror, it was her mother's face she saw. Having surgery on her eyelids, she explained, was symbolic of her commitment to grow through this transition in midlife and to stay open to possibilities. Understanding the unconscious intention behind her decision made this woman's experience richly rewarding.

What Do You Hope to Get or Gain from the Surgery?

Whether the patient's goal is expressed as "I want myself back" or "I want the outside to reflect my inside," being able to give voice to those desires and putting them into a meaningful context will help her achieve what she wants. Since ritual reflects the answers to larger questions, the work the patient puts into articulating her wants, desires, and her vision of life postsurgery is very important. For many women, building an altar before surgery as a way of clarifying these desires and then using the altar as the surgery begins will become a means of a greater healing and self-articulation.

Once again, patients who see their surgery as a means to an end—such as a better job, a new relationship, or as a way of "fixing" some aspect of their life—are likely to be disappointed. We try to discourage these patients from moving forward on this basis.

What Are Your Ambivalent Voices Saying—The Ones That Argue That You Shouldn't Have Surgery?

Confronting the cultural messages all of us absorb and acknowledging our own ambivalences even as we move forward with surgery will increase awareness. Many patients will talk about the money they are spending—whether they feel guilty about spending "money on themselves" or spending money "on something so unnecessary." They worry about the risks of surgery, whether it's about undergoing anesthesia or experiencing a less-than-satisfactory result. And they worry about how others will perceive their decision.

Sometimes patients will discover that the ambivalence they may feel about the surgery is connected to something else entirely, such as needing to please others or worrying about being thought of as shallow or vain. One woman, at the age of sixty, confessed that she worried that her facelift would somehow "erase all the experiences I've had or would appear to be a way of denying that I lived the life I have or made the choices I did." It turned out that she was echoing what her ex-husband had said once he'd heard that she was considering surgery. Women sometimes confess that despite their positive feelings about their surgery, they feel that somehow they are "giving in" or "capitulating" to the tough standards our culture imposes on aging women. These negative feelings may coexist with the positive conviction that altering the body is empowering and fulfilling.

This aspect of the counseling is less about reconciling ambivalences than it is about getting in touch with all of the feelings, positive and negative, about wanting surgery. The goal is integrating the self and resolving inner conflict. In addition, becoming aware of the negative and self-critical "whispering" voices greatly reduces the chances that those voices will sabotage the healing process later.

Ritual disclosure of the hidden aspects of a patient's presurgical thoughts has been invaluable to me as a physician, time and time again. Too often as surgeons, we tend to concern ourselves only with the logistics of preparedness before an operation, asking only whether the patient has realistic expectations, are her lab values normal, is her transportation to and from the hospital arranged, among other things. Although these are admittedly important concerns, they are not the only factors that will affect the outcome of the surgery.

The patient's hidden or less conscious expectations and fears, her inner story about the operation and its outcome, are every bit as significant but more difficult to discover. One woman came in to have a facelift at precisely the same age her mother had hers, and her expectations about the surgery were very much shaped by her mother's negative experience. These often hidden inner stories can affect both the surgery and the recovery, and to this end, the dream journal and the presurgical ritual disclosure are not only important tools for increasing the patient's conscious awareness but invaluable for me as the surgeon as I prepare for the operation.

Is There Pressure on You to Proceed with the Surgery?

There are many different pressures on women to look younger or different, and sorting out how much pressure a woman is feeling and who is exerting it is important as well. Women who choose surgery in the hopes of pleasing someone else—and it doesn't really matter who that someone else is—aren't likely to experience change or, for that matter, satisfaction.

Because surgery is a serious undertaking, it's very important that the patient really is doing it for herself and that she is willingly taking on the responsibility. Sometimes the pressure can be subtle, coming from a need to belong or fit in, which can be a destructive thing when it comes to surgery. Botox parties are one thing; undergoing surgery because your friends and buddies are doing it is quite another. Not that long ago, two women—a sister and a sister-in-law of one of my patients—came in seeking abdominoplasties after my patient had successfully had one at the age of fifty-two. The fifty-two-year-old had the procedure to celebrate the last of her children going off to college. Her surgery was a success in every way and she was thrilled with how she looked and felt. Her sister, who was slightly younger, came in wanting the same procedure, and she, too, came through it successfully. The sister-in-law, though, had a very different mind-set and she was nervous and distracted before her surgery; despite her denials, she seemed afraid of both the procedure and the recovery. Of the three, it was this last patient who had complications and who was, I suspect, persuaded by the two other women to go forward.

Making sure that you fully understand why you are undertaking surgery is key to both your recovery and satisfaction with the results.

How Do Your Loved Ones—Partner, Spouse, Family, Friends—Feel About Your Surgery?

All rites and ritual depend on communal support, and the ones created for the surgical process are no different. We encourage our patients to be open with those who constitute their immediate community and to make every effort to involve them. In our experience, patients who are surrounded by loving and supportive friends and family who want to be part of the transformation will benefit the most. Conversely, patients who aren't as fully supported and who may internalize the critical attitudes of others will not do as well.

What Do You Envision for Your Life After Surgery?

This is less a question about what the surgery will achieve in literal terms than it is about the patient's appreciation and understanding of the surgery as a turning point in his or her life. The rituals we will help the patient create are meant to honor and celebrate that turning point in all of its aspects, as a leaving behind of the past and as a journey into the future. One patient's ritual reenacted the psychological process she wished to complete after suffering a long illness. She put all the photographs of herself during her illness as well as cards and letters she received into a suitcase and decorated it with images of rebirth as well as that of a woman shedding her skin. We threw the suitcase into a hospital Dumpster as part of the rite. One woman symbolically let go of her negative experience of giving birth by putting her journals and notes into a locked box and giving me the key. Other women have focused on the road ahead of them as a new path, and have used symbols of renewal—acorns, flowers, or a picture of the dawn—to make their ritual more meaningful. Some women use their own writing—poetry or journal entries—or that of others as a way of describing and envisioning their postsurgical life more fully.

Approaches to Consciousness

Keeping a dream journal can increase a patient's awareness before surgery, and it is, for many, a new and rewarding experience. Following the model proposed by Carl Jung at the beginning of the twentieth century, we understand dreams to be the repository not just of the unconscious psyche—the experiences we have repressed, images and perceptions we have not fully absorbed from our real-life experiences, raw but unprocessed feelings we have experienced through our bodies—but of universal and archetypal parts of the collective unconscious that we have not yet integrated into the consciousness of the self. As Jung wrote, he "who looks outside, dreams . . . who looks inside, awakens." Because dreams are associative (as opposed to rational or logical), they are filled with images and connection that go beyond the "reality" our waking mind knows.

It's been noted that, in the course of Western history, even as initiatory processes became less conscious and less embodied, they nonetheless remained in dreams and fantasies. Clarissa Pinkola Estés has identified certain types of dreams—the heart-pounding, wake-us-up-in-the-middle-of-the-night dreams—that she believes occur when an initiation is imminent. She describes an initiation as a "psychic change from one level of knowing and behavior to another more mature or more energetic level of knowledge" and notes that initiations occur throughout life, to those who haven't yet experienced their first life passages as well as to those she calls veterans. "No matter how old a woman becomes," she says, "there are more ages, more stages, more 'first times' awaiting her."[4] Sometimes these dreams are of marauders or "dark men." They can serve to shake up the psyche, she writes, when the self has become too complacent, or they can be wake-up calls to increase consciousness.[5]

Not surprisingly, anxious dreams about the surgery or the part of the body that is about to be altered are common, and often prove to be a wellspring of psychic connection. Keeping a dream journal is a creative process that permits a woman to begin to explore the unconscious thoughts that connect to her surgery in a safe environment. Concerns and feelings that would otherwise remain hidden from view are brought out into the open by journaling and can be discussed with the counselor. Even reading over your own journal at home can be deeply revealing.

Dream Incubation: A Conscious Process at Work

Throughout human history, dreams have been used for guidance and healing. The ancient Greeks had temples dedicated to the god of medicine, Asclepius, where men and women would sequester themselves in search of health. Rites of purification were performed to render the supplicant immaculate and render him or her open to the power of the god. Asclepius and his daughter, Hygeia, or the goddess of health, were closely associated with the Earth Mother and her powers of regeneration; the temples dedicated to them were located on sacred mountains—often prone to earthquakes—and near streams, signifying the juncture of death/destruction and life/rebirth. These sacred sites were places of dream incubation where insight and healing would come in the form of dreams, thought to be bestowed by Asclepius himself.

On our own continent, many Native American peoples such as the Ojibwa of the Great Lakes expanded their use of dream incubation to include formation of the self. Adolescents on the cusp of adulthood would embark upon a dream or vision quest into the wilderness as a rite of passage into adulthood and would fast and pray until the anticipated dream was received. The dream was understood to contain guidance about the life path as well as revelations about latent personal talents. The youth would then return to the community, now a responsible adult, ready to apply and share his or her gifts for the benefit of the community.

Dreams are still potential sources of healing and wisdom since they are repositories of the parts of our stories—whether they are stories of the body, the self, or both—hidden from view during the light of day. As Edith Stillwold, a Jungian therapist, writes, "A dream is an event that captures the body, the imagination, and the soul. That is, the senses record the experience in sound and sight, often accompanied by subtle movement of the body; the imagination provides the images, symbols, and story; and the psyche or soul activates the energy to produce the dream."[6] Dreams may also function as a kind of "brainstorming," permitting the dreamer to express or try out new ideas or connections from the information accumulated in memory.

Dream incubation can be practiced and the ability to remember dreams enhanced. Although a forgotten art in our culture, learning from our dreams is natural and neither esoteric nor difficult, and often happens automatically and unconsciously when we fall asleep with a problem in mind. How often have we heard a friend with a problem or a pending decision say, "Let me sleep on it"? Asking a question before you go to sleep is one way to hear your own voice as well as signals from the body and the mind that you are too preoccupied to hear during the day. These signals resonate at night when your muscles and mental chatter are still.

To consciously incubate a dream, simply hold your thoughts or associations in your mind as you prepare for sleep. Relax and ask yourself to have and clearly remember a dream that reveals the questions or thoughts you have about surgery, or the concerns you have about the surgical experience or its outcome. Keep a journal or paper and a pen by your bedside. In the morning, record any dreams you remember or thoughts you have upon waking for later reflection. What you remember and think may be obvious and directly stated or seem opaque or even meaningless, but trust that the process is working. Try to bring whatever insights you have garnered from your dreams and thoughts into the light, and think about how you can use them in your waking life. This last step may require courage and self-discipline to bring what was formerly hidden into the conscious present.

I frequently use dream incubation with my breast cancer patients. If a woman has two reconstructive options, an implant reconstruction or a TRAM flap, or if she has to decide between a mastectomy and a lumpectomy, I will always tell her to make a decision before she goes to sleep and then watch how her inner psyche, in the form of dreams and early waking thought, deals with the decision she has made. If she awakens with the thought "I should not do this!" then she's made the wrong decision. I'm also not surprised to learn that my patients are aware of the fact that they have involved lymph nodes or metastases before they are revealed by a medical work-up. We often have much more unconscious information about our own bodies than we give ourselves credit for with our conscious minds.

Altars and Ritual Process

Creating an altar in the weeks before surgery which will then be used as part of a ritual in the operating room is another way of opening up the conscious process. While some patients already have altars in their homes for reflection and meditation and thus are familiar with the process of creating sacred space, others discover it for the first time. In all cases, though, since the altar is being created for a specific purpose—clarifying intention and ritualizing the act of submitting to surgery—what emerges is full of symbolic content.

An altar that uses images and symbols of the self both in the past and the present as well as images of the self in the future can help make the process of physical and spiritual transformation more concrete. We encourage patients to bring images of mentors, guides, or deities to whom they have a strong connection or from whom they have garnered inspiration. These can be images or objects representative or symbolic of real people in their lives, or of guardians from different spiritual traditions. Alternatively, using symbols and images to represent the life path—past, present, and the postsurgical future— can also help the patient attain greater clarity. It's not unusual for patients to incorporate images of snakes, butterflies, or frogs—all of which symbolize rebirth and transformation—on their altars.

We ask that the patient begin by visualizing the altar she wishes to create and to explore the connections between the objects she decides to place on it and her hopes and dreams for her life after surgery. Each person will approach creating her altar distinctively, using personal as well as universal objects and symbols, and we stress that there is no "right" way to create an altar. One woman who understood her surgery as a journey into wholeness, leaving behind the fragments of her unhappy past self, placed photographs of herself as a girl and an adolescent to symbolize the past on the left side of her altar; she surrounded these photographs with eggshells because, as she put it, she had so little confidence that she felt that "she'd been walking on eggshells all of her life." In the middle of the altar were photographs of her husband and children, as well as dried flowers from her garden, symbolizing the growth of connections she had experienced during the adult years of her life. On the right side of her altar were symbols of the future she felt the surgery would open her to: pieces of crystal for insight and self-awareness, rocks for strength, postcards of blue skies, fluffy clouds, and calm waters.

We often encourage patients to illustrate the stories of the body as well as the inner story of the life transition at hand on their altars. One woman illustrated her life path as a winding "stream" of sand that ended abruptly with a pile of pebbles. When asked to explain it, she said that the pebbles—which looked more like a miniature barrier or wall than anything else—represented menopause and "drying up." Simply putting her feelings into three-dimensional form on the altar allowed her to begin exploring the loss of feminity she associated with menopause.

Like all ritual actions, creating an altar opens a door or gateway to seeing what is already there; altar building doesn't create mystery but only reveals it.

At the time of the surgery, the altar is placed on a prep table or Mayo Stand; the patient sometimes brings in an altar cloth, and we play music during the ritual. Sometimes the altar will contain just artwork, or religious objects, or images and objects that the patient feels connect her to the larger community, the world, or the universe. Altars can be simple—a grouping of shells (symbolizing the oceans), feathers (lightness of being or flight), and flowers (emergence and rebirth)—or complex, since this activity is more about process than it is about achieving an end result.

Julia's Story: The Impact of Transformational Healing

As she tells it, the experience of her surgery was "one of the most incredible and uplifting experiences" of her life, and one that had an "immense and powerful impact" on her well-being and health. While the life passages Julia experienced were perhaps more complicated and painful than some others—she had survived breast cancer, had an unreconstructed mastectomy, and then tried unsuccessfully to conceive and then bear a child—her experience nonetheless has universal application.

Both the experience of cancer and over two years of fertility treatments had left Julia at a low point in her life; she felt, as she puts it, "overwhelming feelings of despair, sadness, and hopelessness." The challenges she had faced took on, for her, a unique form: "The biggest impact I felt was a complete disconnection to any femininity and sense of feeling like a woman. In my mind, I had failed at the 'normal' effort of a woman having a baby. I'd lost a breast to cancer, and despite the conscious acceptance of knowing intellectually that this physical change had nothing to do with my essential femininity, I felt a sense of loss and disconnect with the sensual and the female that is embodied in the breast. I felt like a person who had been cheated and victimized—not how I had ever felt before or a place I'd ever been."

Julia decided to move forward by having breast reconstruction, though she acknowledged, as she puts it, that the "surgery itself wasn't a cure-all to regaining my femininity. What *was* a major step was making a choice to create my sense of femininity anew. I wanted to approach this surgery in a holistic way, taking into account all that it meant in my life and what I wanted my life to be." She began preparing for her surgery six weeks ahead of the scheduled date, meeting with a therapist every two weeks. Each of the sessions delved into Julia's sense of loss as well as her hopes and dreams for the future. She built an altar symbolizing the significance of the surgery in her life, with images and objects that had emotional and symbolic resonance for her. Rocks from significant places in her life—from her family's farm, her mother's birthplace, from Lake Tahoe where she and her family have a home and which they consider a place closest to heaven. A photograph of herself as a young girl of five or six when she had what Julia called "a world of dreams in my head," one of which was of being a beautiful and feminine woman. A photograph of her with her husband and her two stepchildren, "the loves of my life." A photograph of herself with her father, whom she describes as "a hugely influential and important person in my life from whom I always wanted approval." Their relationship today is a wonderful and strong one, but it wasn't always so. Two sets of rosary beads given to her by friends—one on the occasion of her mastectomy and the other for her reconstruction. Although Julia isn't Catholic, each friend reported that she "knew" the beads were meant to help her healing and health. All the other objects on the altar related directly to the cancer and the reconstruction.

In addition to creating an altar and writing prayers to be read at the altar before surgery, Julia asked her circle of friends and family for prayer support; some one hundred fifty friends, family members, and coworkers prayed and sent positive thoughts and energy to her during the operation. The operation itself was preceded by a prayer ceremony conducted by a minister and witnessed by Julia's mother and husband. The ritual performed in front of her altar before the start of surgery enacted her desire to regain her wholeness and femininity.

The surgery was a technical success but the transformation went far beyond the physical reconstruction of her breast. Julia's own words best capture what this moment of transformation was like and how it connected to her surgery: "I have regained the sense of femininity I felt disconnected from. Instead of feeling victimized by all of the challenges connected to my health, the rituals helped me define what I wanted to create in my life from the surgery and beyond. The altar I created for the surgery has since been expanded to include objects and symbols of the femininity I feel every day, and I've continued to perform rituals of thankfulness for my wholeness as a woman. Finally, my willingness to share the transformational process, along with my dreams and desires, had a tremendous effect on the people in my life. They became part of the process and were themselves empowered and made whole by the help they could give me."

Transformation Without Surgery

It goes without saying that life passages *can* be forded and a change from one level of being and awareness to another *can* be achieved without surgery, though I would say categorically that, for it to be a true rite of passage, it must involve both the mind and the body. Mindfulness and consciousness are still key to the process, as they are to the ritual initiation surgery represents. There must also be a hiatus in life's rhythms—a "before" and an "after" experienced both physically and psychologically—that helps the individual achieve transformation. We all know women who, facing a turning point in their lives, use their energies to propel themselves in a different direction and succeed, on their own, in transforming themselves inside and out. Some women will seek a therapist's help, while others manage to forge a new path on their own. Most of these stories will include "wake-up calls" or moments of recognition of an event or events that signal a life transition and spark a determination in the individual to transform herself spiritually and physically.

My coauthor's story is one of transformation without surgery, and while the details are singular, there is much about the story that is typical of the midlife transition. It serves as a reminder that there is more than one pathway to inner and outer transformation at a moment of crisis.

Peg delivered her only daughter by C-section just a month before her thirty-ninth birthday. It was a turning point—something which, to this day, she considers the most significant event of her life. The transition into motherhood eclipsed whatever life passage she might have experienced going into her forties; she had little time to focus on anything other than her small child and her career as a writer. Much to her surprise, motherhood became her primary way of defining herself. "I did other things, of course—I worked, I had a husband, friends—but I really thought of myself first and foremost as a mother. I never fully lost all the weight I gained during pregnancy, but I didn't really care since I was never all that invested in my body to begin with." When she was forty-seven and her daughter eight, her marriage of sixteen years ended. She embarked on raising her child alone: "My world, at that point, became small by choice. I made the deliberate decision not to date because I thought the damage caused by divorce had to do with the introduction of new people into the household. I defined myself by mothering and work—and all the other selves I used to be gradually disappeared from view."

Life went on, and Peg considered herself content. Then, the year she turned fifty—which coincided with her daughter's going to middle school and becoming increasingly independent—the uterine fibroids she'd had since pregnancy suddenly flared up. Her belly swelled to the size of a twenty-week pregnancy. "I knew my inner babe—the part of me that had been flirty and funny and sexy—had been put on hold, but when this happened, that part of me simply disappeared. I stopped thinking of myself as a sexual creature, let alone a sexy woman." She went from doctor to doctor, all of whom recommended surgery. Ultimately, she decided not to have the surgery, hoping that the onset of menopause would shrink the fibroids in due course. That didn't happen on schedule, either: "It went on for years, and I just gave up on my body and looking good. Even though I didn't recognize it at the time, my belly became an excuse for not exercising or watching what I ate. Since I couldn't do anything about my belly—there wasn't any way of changing the distension—I felt I couldn't do anything at all. And so I didn't. I was looking away from the crossroads I'd reached—my own middle age and my daughter's adolescence. At the same time, the heavier I got, the worse I felt. I didn't realize it, but I was just treading water, moving forward through life."

The crisis came when Peg was fifty-five and her daughter, now 16, went to a pre-college program: "Suddenly I realized the future was almost here, and I wasn't ready for it. It was as though I woke up one morning and discovered I was middle-aged overnight. My daughter would be going off to college in a few years and what would happen to me? Was I going to end up eating alone, surrounded by my cats, sipping wine every night? I woke up to the fact that I had to get to the other side."

The crisis galvanized her. She began by connecting with other women who were single and childless or who had made the transition when their children left home. She started keeping a journal and built an altar to symbolize her intention to change. She asked herself something she hadn't asked herself in years—"What is it that I want for myself now and in the future, separate from my role as a mother?"—and, most important, she began to pay attention to her body with a program of exercise and diet: "I looked at myself in the mirror and saw a woman who hadn't exercised in years, whose gait was stiff, and whose body was wide and fleshy. My belly was stretched and distended, to be sure, but that wasn't all I saw. I realized that what I was seeing in the mirror was symbolic of what had happened to me. I had always taken care of myself as a matter of pride, and somehow that had gotten lost. I knew I had to find the 'me' buried in my body—the 'me' who felt good when she looked good, who liked touching and being touched, who enjoyed being a woman with a man. I knew a crash diet—like the ones I used to go on when I was young—wouldn't work. I needed to make getting in shape reflect the process I was going through, and it had to be a long-term commitment."

Slowly but surely, Peg incorporated exercise into her life: "I felt that taking my body in hand was symbolic of taking control of my life. I started out being able to do all of two crunches—much to my daughter's amusement—and built up to twenty over a course of weeks. I started working out in the gym, in small increments. I first ran half a mile, then a mile, and then increased the pace. I made myself conscious of what I was eating, instead of just eating because the food was there. And I kept asking myself what it was that I wanted. I bought a scale after three weeks of working out, knowing I had lost weight, and jumped off of it, screaming, when I looked down and saw what I actually weighed. The number was symbolic of how lost I'd gotten."

The stronger Peg got—she was walking two or three miles a day, doing two hundred crunches—the better and more focused she felt. "It wasn't just losing weight but feeling more centered than I had in a very long time. I started looking forward into my future, feeling more hopeful about my life than I had in a long time. I started seeing my body in a more positive and less critical way. I started working on being open to the world in ways I hadn't been in a long time." She celebrated losing twenty pounds by buying herself blue jeans and made plans to visit the man she'd dated in college over the Fourth of July weekend, after her daughter left for her summer program.

It's now been two years since Peg saw what she needed to see. She's lost almost forty pounds, and exercise and eating right have become part of the routine of her life. She has remarried—to the man she loved in college and whom she saw that Fourth of July weekend—and is ready for her child to go off to college. She looks very different now than she did several years ago but, most important, she feels very different: "I changed almost everything about how I looked to reflect the new path I was taking. I cut my hair short, streaked it, finally pierced my ears, and stopped wearing nothing but black. I had a closet full of black clothes then, and now I wear things that reveal me instead of covering me. I'm still making peace with my body in its middle-aged form and I've been lucky to have a cheering squad—my new husband and my daughter—who are proud of the work I've accomplished. I feel vibrant and sexy without denying that the body I live in has more than a few miles on it. I've even begun to make peace with my belly and take pride in how I've been able to change it without feeling that I have to make it flat or perfect. I'm learning to turn off those self-critical voices, and as a result, I'm seeing what I call the midlife journey differently."

Peg hasn't ruled out surgery, saying that she probably plans on getting her eyelids done in the next few years but that she needs to think about doing more: "I'm still learning to listen to myself. I think

I'll know the answer to whether or not to pursue cosmetic surgery when I'm ready. For now, I'm just happy to be in a new place, on a new path. So much has changed in my life and is still changing that I have a sense of actually being reborn in a very real way."

I don't think it's an accident that Peg's belly became, at this point in her life, the most "storied" part of her body—closely connected both to her motherhood and her sense of herself as a woman.

It's important to remember that while cosmetic surgery can be a tool for true transformation, it isn't the only tool, and that if the surgery isn't accompanied by conscious process, it's not likely to accomplish the life transition or passage you are facing. Spiritual growth depends on fully integrating the self—body and soul. That means that no matter which path you choose to follow—with surgery or without—you must first learn to listen to all the stories both your body and your spirit tell.

Ensuring Conscious Process

While the techniques we have developed are, in many ways, unique to a surgical practice, there are basic principles and approaches that can be used by any woman who has decided on cosmetic surgery as a tool for transformation. Conscious process begins with awareness of the surgery itself and then fans out from there into an exploration of the personal story behind the choice to have surgery.

The Procedure
Make sure you are fully informed about the procedure you have decided on, and research it to make sure you know precisely what is involved. Familiarize yourself with both the benefits of the surgery and its possible negatives. If you can, network to find women who have undergone the procedure you are considering, and learn about

their experiences. If you can't, this should be one of the first questions you ask your physician: whether you may contact his or her former patients.

The Physician

There are really two aspects to choosing your doctor: The first has to do with his or her credentials and expertise and the second with your level of comfort and connection to him or her. You should check that your doctor is board certified and, as a precaution, contact the state medical board to see if there are any complaints outstanding or whether the physician has been subject to disciplinary action. Ask your doctor how many times he or she has performed this specific procedure and ask to see photographs—"before" and "after"—of the procedure with what the doctor thinks are "average" results. Remind yourself as you talk to the doctor that much of what constitutes a "good" or "great" result is highly subjective. Ask if your surgeon is willing to let you call former patients, both those who have had good outcomes and those who have had complications. Discuss possible complications with your doctor as well as side effects, and make sure that you see photographs of postoperative scars.

Now comes the second part, which is different from an appraisal of the physician's technical expertise. Ask yourself how you feel about him or her. How forthcoming was he or she in answering your questions? How complete was the information you were given? Do you feel he or she understands your goals in undertaking surgery?

Your Job as a Patient

Because surgery is a serious undertaking, you need to make sure you are being straightforward and realistic about your role, as well as your expectations. Have you read all the information you were given about preparing for the procedure, the procedure itself, and recovering? Have you asked all the questions you need to? Are there areas you don't fully understand?

Have you been totally forthright with your doctor about your medical history, medical problems, previous surgeries, as well as all medications and supplements you are taking? This includes not just prescription drugs but over-the-counter medicines, herbals, recreational drugs, cigarettes, and alcohol.

Did you allow enough time for recovery, and do you have adequate emotional and physical support in the postoperative period? Is anyone picking you up from surgery and staying with you the first night?

Are you willing and able to deal with a complication should it occur? Complications involve your health, your emotions, and your finances, and you need to consider all of these factors.

Explore the Connections Between the Surgery and Your Life

Work on asking yourself the questions we ask our transformational surgery patients on pages 112–119. Most of all, examine the link between your desire for surgery and what is going on in your life now. You can make the process more conscious by journaling or altar-building and through honest discussions with loved ones and friends. If the body part you are considering changing could speak to you, what would it say? And how would you answer?

Face the Surgery and the Recovery Directly

Listen to yourself. What, if any, of the aspects of the surgery make you unsure or nervous? Have you prepared yourself for your recovery? What is it that you want from the surgery, and do you think it can be achieved? Ask yourself honestly whether you feel pressured to do what you are doing.

Plan on giving yourself time for healing and recovery. Do not catapult yourself back into your life as though nothing has happened; something *has* happened.

Toward a Vision of Wholeness

When we are small children, drawing a picture of the self is a straight-forward process: Grab some crayons and paper and the picture that emerges is the exterior self, among trees, flowers, and clouds, or perhaps surrounded by siblings, parents, friends, or pets. "This is me!" the picture proclaims, with a confidence rarely, if ever, matched by an adult faced with the same task. What *is* the self, after all? It isn't just that exterior—eyes, nose, mouth, hair, and all the rest—but something more complicated, a brew concocted of life experience: the thoughts we think and have thought, the emotions we feel and have felt, the people we've loved as well as the ones we've lost, the places we've been and those we dream of getting to, the pain and pleasure etched in colors and line. To picture all the stories that make up the self, we would need much more than a box of crayons.

In these pages, I've talked about cosmetic surgery as a powerful tool that can be used as a way of transforming the self in the broadest sense, both inside and out. But, like all powerful instruments of change, cosmetic surgery can be used to great benefit or detriment, and I would be the first to admit that as surgery becomes more and more of a commodity to be bought and sold, the potential downside is already clear.

While I have argued that cosmetic surgery can help integrate and give an embodied voice to the self in a new stage of life, there is no question that it can also render the self inauthentic in ways that go far beyond the surface. Trends in cosmetic surgery that are depicted on television, such as those that give a person "a famous face," obliterating whatever individuality the patient has, fall into this category, as do surgeries that seek to erase ethnic characteristics that are part of the person's roots and history. Michael Jackson's surgeries are perhaps the most notorious and radical examples but they are, unfortunately, not unique. The opening of Asian eyes, the narrowing of African-

American features, as well as the surgery that tries to change a face or feature into that of a celebrity share much in common: These surgeries are efforts to hide and deny both the story of the self as it is expressed in the body and to eradicate the storied aspects of the body itself. At the very least, undergoing these surgeries is an act of self-effacement. In my opinion, these surgeries are a product of a patient's misguided efforts to alter him- or herself in unhealthy ways and a surgeon's willingness to collude in the effort.

Surgeries that deny the integrity of the body and the self in basic ways—ones that focus only on the surface—are also more damaging and detrimental than whatever fleeting satisfaction they may give patients. Take the example of celebrities who have chosen to stop the clock at age twenty-five, ultimately rendering them stiffened and stretched parodies of themselves thirty years later. A facelift that tries to make a patient look decades younger than she is will not only make her skin look stretched but will lay waste to how her face, in its natural state, was expressive and animated, since it changes the movement of muscle and ligaments as they attach to the bone. It will alter the appearance forever, so much so that the person is rendered, in a real sense, no longer recognizable as herself. This is clearly not a trend any one of us would recognize as healthy or desirable, since life isn't and shouldn't be static in that sense, nor should surgery change a person's basic expressions, as I remind patients who come in with twenty-year-old pictures of themselves to show me what they want. In these cases, cosmetic surgery is used to deny the evolution of the self, the stages of life, and the passage of time—a perspective that manages to be literally self-effacing, unhealthy, and finally self-defeating all at once. There is no fountain of youth, after all; in the end, all of us will end up old, no matter what we do to try to intervene in the process.

These are all examples of surgeries that are efforts to escape the perceived confines of the self and attempt to supplant the self's true stories—contained within the body—with a wholly different set of stories that have no connection to the individual. They are a product of dangerous wishful thinking—"If I could look like her, then I could be her and live her life "—and have nothing at all to do with human transformation or happiness. They are substitutes for coping with the human condition.

They stand in marked contrast to consciously realized surgeries, which seek to integrate the self, body, and spirit.

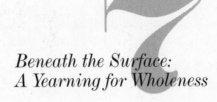

Beneath the Surface:
A Yearning for Wholeness

A few years ago, a television documentary was made about one of my patients, the breast surgery she'd elected, and the rituals she had created for her operation. Although the show ended up being aired for two years, the producers were disappointed at first that the changes made to my patient's body were so subtle. They wanted something more dramatic and easily identifiable as "life-changing"—a "before" and "after" that needed no voice-over, a bold new cup size that was proof of transformation—even though every word my patient spoke on film made it clear that her surgery marked an important turning point in her life.

While a more radical makeover might have made for more sensational television, it wouldn't have altered what my patient felt her surgery would achieve: a sense of wholeness. Surgery had allowed her to recast her story of self because she had chosen it with purpose and consciousness, which were heightened by the rituals she'd helped create. The submission to the surgery, the discomfort and scarring, and the period of recovery transformed both her body and mind at once. The physical change in her body—the aspect most visible to the outside observer—was only a part of what had taken place.

In this book, I've suggested that many of my patients choose to undergo cosmetic surgery to heal and transform themselves, to become whole in the anticipation or the wake of a life passage or transition. The yearning for wholeness—the desires for a coherent self and for connection to something larger outside the self—was, throughout the course of much of human history, satisfied by rites that involved both the individual and his or her community. Contemporary psychoanalysts, therapists, and sociologists have suggested that, in the absence of meaningful rites, human beings will seek other ways of filling that yearning for wholeness with a range of behaviors, both healthy and not.[1] Recent scientific literature gives even more credence to that point of view by suggesting that the need for ritualistic behavior, as well as its effects, may well be biologically hardwired into the human species.[2]

It shouldn't surprise us, then, that at those moments of life transition when our need for rite is most acute—when we embark on a new stage of life, when our children leave home, or when we experience severe loss—many of us will find our own ways of satisfying that need. I believe that cosmetic surgery has become one of them.

This isn't to say that I think cosmetic surgery should be seen as the preferred or only pathway to spiritual growth, particularly since it's clear that some women will choose surgery in order to look away from life crises and issues of self, rather than confronting them. But it does mean that we need to reshape our discussions about cosmetic surgery as a cultural phenomenon to better understand the motivations of women who consciously choose it for themselves, on the one hand, and to actively discourage women who use it as a form of denial or avoidance, on the other.

The need for a new discussion seems particularly urgent since, as a cultural fact and phenomenon, cosmetic surgery is here to stay. It seems likely that as greater numbers of us decide to undergo surgery, it will become more the norm and some of the moral objections to it—particularly those having to do with vanity and self-absorption—will become faint background noise, just as the objections to makeup did some eighty years ago. Young adults are already inclined to see the body as a canvas for self-expression, as the high percentage of those who have piercing and tattoos attest,[3] and as they come of age, societal hesitations about altering the body through surgery may, over time, simply disappear.

This is all the more reason that doctors and patients alike should address the mind-body connection as they work together to reshape the body. The surgical process needs to be kept center stage, an antidote to the sugarcoating preferred by television and advertising, which suggests that it is "a casual beauty treatment"[4] or a commodity to be bought and sold. Women who are considering surgery would be wise to understand it in the context of their lives and their own inner stories, remembering that while surgery can produce extraordinary physical changes, those alterations alone are unlikely to result in contentment or happiness unless the inner story changes as well. Women who turn to cosmetic surgery as a form of denial—of self or life circumstance—or who look away from or minimize the seriousness of the process should be actively discouraged from going through with it.

If that happens, cosmetic surgery may achieve its potential as a tool of integration, one that can, when used consciously and with agency, help each patient realize herself in wholeness. Perhaps, at that point, the distinction between "reconstructive" and "cosmetic" surgeries will no longer matter, and the invisible but palpable divide in my waiting room will just disappear.

ACKNOWLEDGMENTS

This book is dedicated to my teachers and friends Kali Ma and Francoise Bourzat, who have reawakened my heart and opened my eyes. To Carole Kammen for her ideas, inspiration, and partnership in this project. To my family, who have taught me to think outside the box and loved me no matter what. To my second family at Women's Plastic Surgery for caring for me and my patients so wonderfully. And finally, to Peg Streep, whose vision, patience, and skill transformed this book from a dream into a reality.

Thanks, too, to Gail Winston, and the staff at HarperCollins.

—*L.B.E.*

Thanks to my friends—most specially Leslie Garisto, Peter Israel, and Lori Stein—for the usual acts of kindness, and to my husband, Craig, for his love and support, and to my daughter, Alexandra, for being my shining light and inspiration.

—*P.S.*

NOTES

Chapter 1
Cosmetic Surgery and the Promise of Transformation

1. Statistics from the American Society of Plastic Surgeons, www.plasticsurgery.org.
2. *People* magazine, June 7, 2004.
3. Grant S. Hamilton III, M.D. "Public Perception of the Terms 'Cosmetic,' 'Plastic,' and 'Reconstructive' Surgery," *Archives of Facial Plastic Surgery*, 6 (2004): 315–320.
4. AARP survey, Roper Starch, January 2001.
5. Joan Jacobs Brumberg, *The Body Project: An Intimate History of American Girls* (New York: VintageBooks, 1997).

Chapter 2
America and Cosmetic Surgery: Loving It, Hating It

1. Kathy Peiss, *Hope in a Jar: The Making of America's Beauty Culture* (New York: Metropolitan Books, 1998), p. 7.
2. Ibid., p. 144.

3. Ibid., pp. 260–262.

4. Elizabeth Haiken, *Venus Envy: A History of Cosmetic Surgery* (Baltimore: The Johns Hopkins University Press, 1997), pp. 17–34.

5. Ibid., p. 98.

6. Ibid., p. 123.

7. Ibid., p. 130.

8. Maureen Dowd, "The Knife Under the Tree," *New York Times*, December 25, 2002, p. A. 23.

9. Phil Rosenthal, "Avert Your Gaze: The Swan Is Back," *Chicago Sun-Times*, October 25, 2004.

10. Barbara Lippert, "The Bad and the Ugly," *Adweek*, May 31, 2004.

11. Simon Dumenco, "Their Bodies, Ourselves," *New York*, October 6, 2003, p. 43.

12. Ruth Shalit, "*Extreme Makeover:* The Truth Behind the Show," *Elle*, January 2004, p. 148.

13. "The War Over Plastic Surgery: Stars Take Sides," *People*, vol. 62, no. 16 (October 18, 2004), p. 60.

14. Natasha Singer, "The New Normal," *W* magazine, November 2004, p. 174.

15. Margaret Olivia Little, "Cosmetic Surgery, Suspect Norms, and the Ethics of Complicity," in *Enhancing Human Traits: Ethical and Social Implications,* edited by Erik Parens (Washington, D.C.: Georgetown University Press, 1998), pp. 162–176.

16. Christine Rosen, "The Democratization of Beauty," *The New Atlantis: A Journal of Technology and Society* (Spring 2004).

17. Ibid.

18. Haiken, op. cit., pp. 300–301.

19. Susan Bordo, *Unbearable Weight: Feminism, Western Culture, and the Body* (Berkeley and Los Angeles: University of California Press, 1993), p. 5.

20. Carl Elliott, *Better than Well: American Medicine Meets the American Dream* (New York: W. W. Norton & Company, 2003), p. 27.

21. Naomi Wolf, *The Beauty Myth: How Images of Beauty Are Used Against Women* (New York: Anchor Books, 1992), p. 232.

22. Ibid., p. 259.

23. Ibid., p. 257.

24. Susan Bordo, "*Braveheart, Babe,* and the Contemporary Body," in *Enhancing Human Traits: Social and Ethical Implications,* edited by Erik Parens (Washington, D.C.: Georgetown University Press, 1998), p. 202.

25. Sheila M. Rothman and David J. Rothman, *The Pursuit of Perfection: The Promise and Perils of Medical Enhancement* (New York: Vintage Books, 2003).

Chapter 3
The Stories the Body Tells

1. Joan Cassell, *The Woman in the Surgeon's Body* (Cambridge, Mass.: Harvard University Press, 1998), p. 17.

2. Ibid., p. 31.

3. Thomas F. Cash, "Cognitive-Behavioral Perspectives on Body Image," in *Body Image: A Handbook of Theory, Research, and Clinical Practice,* edited by Thomas F. Cash and Thomas Pruzinsky (New York and London: The Guilford Press, 2002), pp. 38–46.

4. Thomas F. Cash and Thomas Pruzinsky, "Integrative Themes on Body-Image Development and Change," in *Body Images: Development, Deviance, and Change,* edited by Thomas F. Cash and Thomas Pruzinsky (New York: The Guilford Press, 1990), p. 40.

5. David W. Kruger, "Psychodynamic Perspectives on Body Image," in *Body Image: A Handbook of Theory, Research, and Clinical Practice*, edited by Thomas F. Cash and Thomas Pruzinsky (New York and London: The Guilford Press, 2002), pp. 30–37.

6. Kathy Davis, *Reshaping the Female Body: The Dilemma of Cosmetic Surgery* (New York: Routledge, 1995), pp. 112–114.

7. See, for example, Francine Shapiro, Ph.D., *EMDR: Eye Movement Desensitization and Reprocessing* (New York: The Guilford Press, 2001); *EMDR: The Breakthrough "Eye Movement" Therapy for Overcoming Anxiety, Stress, and Trauma* (New York: Basic Books, 1997); *EMDR as an Integrative Psychotherapy Approach* (Washington, D.C.: American Psychological Association, 2002), and Candace Pert, Ph.D., *Molecules of Emotion: The Science Behind Mind-Body Medicine* (New York: Scribner, 1997).

8. Antonio Damasio, *The Feeling of What Happens: Body and Emotion in the Making of Consciousness* (San Diego and New York: Harcourt, Inc., 1999), p. 145.

9. Ibid., p. 145.

Chapter 4
Cosmetic Surgery and Rites of Passage

1. My understanding of rites of passage and their meaning and significance is drawn primarily from the following sources: Arnold Van Gennep, *The Rites of Passage*; Mircea Eliade, *Rites and Symbols of Initiation: The Mysteries of Birth and Rebirth*; Mircea Eliade, *The Sacred and the Profane: The Nature of Religion*; Victor Turner, *The Ritual Process: Structure and Anti-Structure*; René Girard, *Violence and the Sacred*; and Joseph Campbell, *The Hero with a Thousand Faces*.

2. Bruce Lincoln, *Emerging from the Chrysalis: Rituals of Women's Initiations* (New York: Oxford University Press, 1991), pp. 94–95.

3. Mircea Eliade, *Rites and Symbols of Initiation: The Mysteries of Birth and Rebirth*, translated by Willard R. Trask (Putnam, Conn.: Spring Publications, 1994), p. 3.

4. Joseph Campbell, *The Hero with a Thousand Faces* (Princeton, N.J.: Princeton University Press, 1972), p. 10.

5. David Cohen, ed., *The Circle of Life: Rituals from the Human Family Album* (San Francisco: HarperSanFrancisco, 1991), p. 70.

6. Eliade, op. cit., p. 134.

7. See particularly C. G. Jung, *Symbols of Transformation* and *Memories, Dreams, and Reflections*.

8. Robert L. Moore, *The Archetype of Initiation: Sacred Space, Ritual Process, and Personal Transformation* (Philadelphia: Xlibris, 2001), p. 39.

9. Eliade, op. cit., pp. 134–135.

10. Andrew Newberg, M.D., Eugene D'Aquill, M.D., Ph.D., and Vince Rause, *Why God Won't Go Away: Brain Science and the Biology of Belief* (New York: Ballantine Books, 2001), pp. 74–75.

11. Michael Meade, introduction to Eliade, op. cit., p. xxii.

12. Judith Viorst, *Necessary Losses: The Loves, Illusions, Dependencies and Impossible Expectations That All of Us Have to Give Up in Order to Grow* (New York: Simon & Schuster, 1986), p. 16.

13. M. Scott Peck, M.D., *The Road Less Traveled: A New Psychology of Love, Traditional Values and Spiritual Growth* (New York: Touchstone, 1978), p. 74.

14. Victor Turner, *The Ritual Process: Structure and Anti-Structure* (New York: Aldine de Gruyter, 1995), p. 94.

15. Robert L. Moore, op. cit., p. 59.

16. *The Essential Rumi*, translated by Coleman Barks (San Francisco: HarperSanFrancisco, 1995), p. 142.

17. Elizabeth Hayt, "Over-40 Rebels with a Cause: Tattooing," *New York Times*, December 22, 2002.

18. Julie Salamon, "Tragedy Pierces the Heart, Memory the Skin," *New York Times*, April 4, 2003, p. 35.

19. Susan Benson, "Inscriptions on the Self: Reflections on Tattooing and Piercing in Contemporary Euro-America," in *Written on the Body: The Tattoo in European and American History*, edited by Jane Caplan (Princeton, N.J.: Princeton University Press, 2000), pp. 234–254.

20. Marion Woodman, *Addiction to Perfection: The Still Unravished Bride* (Toronto, Can.: Inner City Books, 1982), p. 29.

21. For example, see Luigi Zoja, *Drugs, Addiction, and Initiation: The Modern Search for Ritual*, translated by Marc E. Romano and Robert Mecurio (Einseidlen, Switzerland: Daimon Verlag, 2000), and *Crossroads: The Quest for Contemporary Rites of Passage*, edited by Louise Carus Mahdi, Nancy Gever Christopher, and Michael Meade (Chicago: Open Court, 1996).

22. Kim Chernin, *The Hungry Self: Women, Eating, and Identity* (New York: HarperPerennial, 1985), p. 166.

23. Ibid., p. 167.

24. Ibid., p. 169.

25. Ginia Bellafante, "When Midlife Seems Just an Empty Plate," *New York Times*, March 9, 2003.

26. Sandra Kronberg, M.S., R.D., C.D.N. and Vicki Paley, C.S.W. B.C.D, "The Seasoning of Age: Contemplating the Impact of Midlife Therapists on Treatment," *Perspective: A Professional Journal of the Renfrew Center Foundation* (Summer 2004), p. 10.

27. Kathryn J. Zerbe, "Eating Disorders in Middle and Late Life: A Neglected Problem," *Primary Psychiatry* (June 2003), p. 82.

28. Karen Conterio and Wendy Lader, Ph.D., *Bodily Harm: The Breakthrough Healing Program for Self-Injurers* (New York: Hyperion Books, 1998), p. 11.

29. Susan Benson, "Inscriptions of the Self: Reflections on Tattoo-

ing and Piercing in Contemporary Euro-America," in *Written on the Body: The Tattoo in European and American History*, edited by Jane Caplan (Princeton, N.J.: Princeton University Press, 2000), p. 246.

30. Katherine A. Phillips, *The Broken Mirror: Understanding and Treating Body Dysmorphic Disorder* (Oxford and New York: Oxford University Press, 1998), p. 95 ff. and pp. 300–301.

31. Katherine A. Phillips, "Body Image and Body Dysmorphic Disorder," in *Body Image: A Handbook*, edited by Thomas F. Cash and Thomas Pruzinsky (New York: The Guilford Press, 2002), p. 314.

32. Katherine A. Phillips, *The Broken Mirror*, pp. 165 and 137.

33. Christina Grof, "Rites of Passage: A Necessary Step Towards Wholeness," in *Crossroads: The Quest for Contemporary Rites of Passage*, op. cit., p. 9.

34. Robert L. Moore, op. cit., pp. 48–49.

Chapter 5
Willing Wounds: Surgery as Catalyst

1. Bernie Siegel, *Love, Medicine and Miracles* (New York: HarperPerennial, 1986), p. 190.

2. Ibid., p. 201.

3. Robert L. Moore, *The Archetype of Initiation: Sacred Space, Ritual Process, and Personal Transformation* (Philadelphia: Xlibris, 2001), pp. 108–112.

4. Thomas Pruzinsky and Milton T. Edgerton, "Body-Image Change in Cosmetic Surgery," in *Body Images: Development, Deviance, and Change*, edited by Thomas F. Cash and Thomas Pruzinsky (New York: The Guilford Press, 1990), pp. 220–221.

5. Ibid., p. 230.

6. Dean Ornish, "Opening Your Heart: Anatomically, Emotionally,

Spiritually," in *Consciousness and Healing: Integral Approaches to Mind-Body Healing*, edited by Marilyn Schlitz and Tina Amorak with Marc S. Mucozzi (St. Louis, Mo.: Elsevier Church Livingstone, 2005), p. 308.

7. Herbert Benson, M.D., *Timeless Healing: The Power and Biology of Belief.* (New York: Fireside Books, 1996), p. 273.

8. Antonio Damasio, *The Feeling of What Happens: Body and Emotion in the Making of Consciousness* (San Diego: Harvest Books, 1999), p. 222.

9. Ibid., pp. 223–225.

10. Susan Saulny, "After Cosmetic Surgery: The Do-Over," *New York Times*, August 4, 2005.

11. Thomas Pruzinsky and Milton T. Edgerton, "Body-Image Change of Cosmetic Plastic Surgery," in *Body Images: Development, Deviances, and Change*, op. cit., pp. 217–236.

Chapter 6
Making the Connection: Ritual and Conscious Process

1. Rachel Naomi Remen, M.D., *Kitchen Table Wisdom: Stories That Heal* (New York: Riverhead Books, 1996), p. 89.

2. Tom Driver, *Liberating Rites: Understanding the Transformative Power of Ritual* (Boulder, Colo.: Westview Press, 1998), p. 93.

3. Natasha Singer, "For You, My Lovely, a Facelift," *New York Times*, December 29, 2005.

4. Clarissa Pinkola Estés, Ph.D., *Women Who Run with the Wolves: Myths and Stories of the Wild Woman Archetype* (New York: Ballantine Books, 1995), p. 68.

5. Ibid., p. 69.

6. Edith Stillwold, Ph.D., "Dream as Story," in *Sacred Stories: A Celebration of the Power of Story to Transform and Heal*, edited

by Charles and Anne Simpkinson (San Francisco: HarperSan-
Francisco, 1993), p. 65.

Chapter 7
Beneath the Surface: A Yearning for Wholeness

1. See, for example, Kim Chernin's *The Hungry Self* and the works
    of Louise Mahdi and Marion Woodman.
2. Andrew Newberg, M.D., Eugene D'Aquili, M.D., Ph.D., and
    Vince Rause, *Why God Won't Go Away: Brain Science and the
    Biology of Belief* (New York: Basic Books, 2001), pp. 86–90.
3. The Mayo Clinic reported in January of 2001 the results of a
    survey of undergraduate students showing that 51 percent had
    body piercings and 23 percent had tattoos. Similarly, a Harris
    Poll found that 35 percent of twenty-five- to twenty-nine-year-
    olds had tattoos.
4. See Natasha Singer, "A Doctor? He *Is* One on TV," *New York
    Times*, March 16, 2006.

SELECTED BIBLIOGRAPHY

Barks, Coleman, trans. *The Essential Rumi*. San Francisco: Harper-SanFrancisco, 1995.

Beckwith, Carole, and Angela Fisher. *African Ceremonies*. New York: Harry N. Abrams, 1999.

Bellafante, Ginia. "When Midlife Seems Just an Empty Plate." *New York Times*, March 9, 2003.

Benson, Herbert, M.D. *Timeless Healing: The Power and Biology of Belief*. New York: Fireside Books, 1996.

Blum, Virginia L. *Flesh Wounds: The Culture of Cosmetic Surgery*. Berkeley and Los Angeles: University of California Press, 2003.

Bordo, Susan. *Unbearable Weight: Feminism, Western Culture, and the Body*. Berkeley and Los Angeles: University of California Press, 1993.

Brumberg, Joan Jacobs. *The Body Project: An Intimate History of American Girls*. New York: Vintage Books, 1997.

Burkert, Walter. *The Creation of the Sacred: Tracks of Biology in Early Religions*. Cambridge, Mass.: Harvard University Press, 1996.

———. *Homo Necans: The Anthropology of Ancient Greek Sacrificial Ritual and Myth*. Translated by Peter Bing. Berkeley: University of California Press, 1983.

Campbell, Joseph. *The Hero with a Thousand Faces*. Princeton, N.J.: Princeton University Press, 1972.

Caplan, Jane, ed. *Written on the Body: The Tattoo in European and American History*. Princeton, N.J.: Princeton University Press, 2000.

Cash, Thomas F. and Thomas Pruzinsky, eds. *Body Image: A Handbook of Theory, Research, and Clinical Practice*. New York and London: The Guilford Press, 2002.

———. *Body Images: Development, Deviance, and Change*. New York: The Guilford Press, 1990.

Cassell, Joan. *The Woman in the Surgeon's Body*. Cambridge, Mass.: Harvard University Press, 1998.

Chernin, Kim. *The Hungry Self: Women, Eating, and Identity*. New York: HarperPerennial, 1985.

Cohen, David, ed. *The Circle of Life: Rituals from the Human Family Album*. San Francisco: HarperSanFrancisco, 1991.

Conterio, Karen, and Wendy Lader, Ph.D. *Bodily Harm: The Breakthrough Healing Program for Self-Injurers*. New York: Hyperion Books, 1998.

Damasio, Antonio. *The Feeling of What Happens: Body and Emotion in the Making of Consciousness*. San Diego and New York: Harcourt, Inc., 1999.

Davis, Kathy. *Dubious Equalities and Embodied Differences: Cultural Studies on Cosmetic Surgery*. Lanham, Md.: Rowman & Littlefield Publishers, 2003.

———. *Reshaping the Female Body: The Dilemma of Cosmetic Surgery*. New York: Routledge, 1995.

Dowd, Maureen. "The Knife Under the Tree." *New York Times*, December 25, 2002.

Driver, Tom. *Liberating Rites: Understanding the Transformative Power of Ritual*. Boulder, Colo.: Westview Press, 1998.

Dumenco, Simon. "Their Bodies, Ourselves," *New York*, October 6, 2003.

Eliade, Mircea. *Rites and Symbols of Initiation: The Mysteries of Birth and Rebirth.* Translated by Willard R. Trask. Putnam, Conn.: Spring Publications, 1994.

———. *The Sacred and the Profane: The Nature of Religion.* Translated by Willard R. Trask. San Diego: Harvest Books, 1987.

Elliott, Carl. *Better than Well: American Medicine Meets the American Dream.* New York: W. W. Norton & Company, 2003.

Estés, Clarissa Pinkola, Ph.D. *Women Who Run with the Wolves: Myths and Stories of the Wild Woman Archetype.* New York: Ballantine Books, 1995.

Etcoff, Nancy. *Survival of the Prettiest: The Science of Beauty.* New York: Anchor Books, 1999.

Favazza, Arnabdo, M.D. *Bodies Under Siege: Self-Mutilation and Body Modification in Culture and Psychiatry.* Baltimore: The Johns Hopkins University Press, 1987, 1996.

Gilman, Sander L. *Creating Beauty to Cure the Soul: Race and Psychology in the Shaping of Aesthetic Surgery.* Durham, N.C.: Duke University Press, 1998.

———. *Making the Body Beautiful: A Cultural History of Aesthetic Surgery.* Princeton, N.J.: Princeton University Press, 1999.

Girard, René. *Violence and the Sacred.* Translated by Patrick Gregory. Baltimore: The Johns Hopkins University Press, 1977.

Haiken, Elizabeth. *Venus Envy: A History of Cosmetic Surgery.* Baltimore: The Johns Hopkins University Press, 1997.

Hamilton, Grant S. III, M.D. "Public Perception of the Terms 'Cosmetic,' 'Plastic,' and 'Reconstructive' Surgery." *Archives of Facial Plastic Surgery,* 6 (2004): 315–320.

Hanh, Thich Nhat. *Essential Writings.* New York: Orbis Books, 2001.

Hayt, Elizabeth. "Over-40 Rebels with a Cause: Tattooing." *New York Times,* December 22, 2002.

Jung, Carl G. *Memories, Dreams, Reflections.* New York: Random House, 1961.

————. *Symbols of Transformation*. Princeton, N.J.: Bollingen, 1956.

Kammen, Carole, and Jodi Gold. *Call to Connection*. Salt Lake City: Commune-A-Key Publishing, 1998.

Lincoln, Bruce. *Emerging from the Chrysalis: Rituals of Women's Initiations*. New York and Oxford: Oxford University Press, 1991.

Lippert, Barbara. "The Bad and the Ugly," *Adweek*, May 31, 2004.

Mahdi, Louise Carus, Nancy Gever Christopher, and Michael Meade, eds. *Crossroads: The Quest for Contemporary Rites of Passage*. Chicago: Open Court, 1996.

Mahdi, Louise Carus, Steven Foster, and Meredith Little, eds. *Betwixt and Between: Patterns of Masculine and Feminine Initiation*. Chicago: Open Court, 1987.

Moore, Robert L.. *The Archetype of Initiation: Sacred Space, Ritual Process, and Personal Transformation*. Philadelphia: Xlibris, 2001.

Newberg, Andrew, M.D., Eugene D'Aquill, M.D., Ph.D., and Vince Rause. *Why God Won't Go Away: Brain Science and the Biology of Belief*. New York: Ballantine Books, 2001.

Parens, Erik, ed. *Enhancing Human Traits: Ethical and Social Implications*. Washington, D.C.: Georgetown University Press, 1998.

Peck, M. Scott, M.D. *The Road Less Traveled: A New Psychology of Love, Traditional Values and Spiritual Growth*. New York: Touchstone, 1978.

Pelletier, Kenneth R. *Mind as Healer, Mind as Slayer: A Holistic Approach to Preventing Stress Disorders*. New York: Dell Publishing, 1977.

Peiss, Kathy. *Hope in a Jar: The Making of America's Beauty Culture*. New York: Metropolitan Books, 1998.

Pert, Candace, Ph.D. *Molecules of Emotion: The Science Behind Mind-Body Medicine*. New York: Scribner, 1997.

Phillips, Katherine A., M.D. *The Broken Mirror: Understanding and Treating Body Dysmorphic Disorder*. Oxford and New York: Oxford University Press, 1998.

Rappaport, Roy. *Ritual and Religion in the Making of Humanity.* Cambridge: Cambridge University Press, 1999.

Remen, Rachel Naomi, M.D., *Kitchen Table Wisdom: Stories That Heal.* New York: Riverhead Books, 1996.

Rosen, Christine. "The Democratization of Beauty." *The New Atlantis: A Journal of Technology and Society* (Spring 2004).

Rosenthal, Phil. "Avert Your Gaze: The Swan Is Back." *Chicago Sun-Times,* October 25, 2004.

Rothman, Sheila M. and David J. Rothman. *The Pursuit of Perfection: The Promise and Perils of Medical Enhancement.* New York: Vintage Books, 2003.

Salamon, Julie. "Tragedy Pierces the Heart, Memory the Skin." *New York Times,* April 4, 2003.

Sarno, John E., M.D. *The Mind-Body Prescription: Healing the Body, Healing the Pain.* New York: Warner Books, 1998.

Saulny, Susan. "After Cosmetic Surgery: The Do-Over." *New York Times,* August 4, 2005.

Schlitz, Marilyn, and Tina Amorak with Marc S. Mucozzi, eds. *Consciousness and Healing: Integral Approaches to Mind-Body Healing.* St. Louis, Mo.: Elsevier Church Livingstone, 2005.

Shalit, Ruth. "Extreme Makeover: The Truth Behind the Show," *Elle,* January 2004.

Shapiro, Francine, Ph.D. *EMDR: Eye Movement Desensitization and Reprocessing.* New York: The Guilford Press, 2001.

———. *EMDR: The Breakthrough "Eye Movement" Therapy for Overcoming Anxiety, Stress, and Trauma.* New York: Basic Books, 1997.

———. *EMDR as an Integrative Psychotherapy Approach.* Washington, D.C.: American Psychological Association, 2002.

Sheehy, Gail. *Passages: Predictable Crises of Adult Life.* New York: E. P. Dutton & Co., 1976.

Siegel, Bernie. *Love, Medicine and Miracles.* New York: HarperPerennial, 1986.

Simpkinson, Charles and Anne Simpkinson, eds. *Sacred Stories: A Celebration of the Power of Story to Transform and Heal.* San Francisco: HarperSanFrancisco, 1993.

Singer, Natasha. "A Doctor? He *Is* One on TV." *New York Times,* March 16, 2006.

———. "For You, My Lovely, a Facelift." *New York Times,* December 29, 2005.

———. "The New Normal." *W* magazine. November 2004.

Sullivan, Deborah A. *Cosmetic Surgery: The Cutting Edge of Commercial Medicine.* New Brunswick, N.J.: Rutgers University Press, 2001.

Turner, Victor. *The Ritual Process: Structure and Anti-Structure.* New York: Aldine de Gruyter, 1995.

Van Gennep, Arnold. *The Rites of Passage.* Translated by Monika B. Vizedom and Gabrielle L. Caffee. Chicago: University of Chicago Press, 1960.

Viorst, Judith. *Necessary Losses: The Loves, Illusions, Dependencies, and Impossible Expectations That All of Us Have to Give Up in Order to Grow.* New York: Simon & Schuster, 1986.

Wolf, Naomi. *The Beauty Myth: How Images of Beauty Are Used Against Women.* New York: Anchor Books, 1992.

Woodman, Marion. *Addiction to Perfection: The Still Unravished Bride.* Toronto, Can.: Inner City Books, 1982.

Zerbe, Kathryn J. "Eating Disorders in Middle and Late Life: A Neglected Problem." *Primary Psychiatry* (June 2003).

Zoja, Luigi. *Drugs, Addiction and Initiation: the Modern Search for Ritual.* Translated by Marc E. Romano and Robert Mecurio. Einseidlen, Switzerland: Daimon Verlag, 2000.

Zweig, Connie. *The Holy Longing: The Hidden Power of Spiritual Yearning.* Boulder, Colo.: Sentient Publications, 2004.

INDEX